Social Determinants of Health

Editors

VINCENT MORELLI
JOEL J. HEIDELBAUGH

PRIMARY CARE:
CLINICS IN OFFICE PRACTICE

www.primarycare.theclinics.com

Consulting Editor
JOEL J. HEIDELBAUGH

December 2023 • Volume 50 • Number 4

ELSEVIER

1600 John F. Kennedy Boulevard • Suite 1800 • Philadelphia, Pennsylvania, 19103-2899

http://www.theclinics.com

PRIMARY CARE: CLINICS IN OFFICE PRACTICE Volume 50, Number 4
December 2023 ISSN 0095-4543, ISBN-13: 978-0-443-18350-8

Editor: Taylor Hayes
Developmental Editor: Nitesh Barthwal

Primary Care: Clinics in Office Practice (ISSN: 0095-4543) is published quarterly by Elsevier Inc., 360 Park Avenue South, New York, NY 10010-1710. Months of issue are March, June, September, and December. Periodicals postage paid at New York, NY and additional mailing offices. Subscription prices are $277.00 per year (US individuals), $629.00 (US institutions), $100.00 (US students), $321.00 (Canadian individuals), $712.00 (Canadian institutions), $100.00 (Canadian students), $379.00 (international individuals), $712.00 (international institutions), and $175.00 (international students). Foreign air speed delivery is included in all *Clinics* subscription prices. All prices are subject to change without notice. POSTMASTER: Send address changes to *Primary Care: Clinics in Office Practice*, Elsevier Periodicals Customer Service, 11830 Westline Industrial Drive, St. Louis, MO 63146. Customer Service Health Sciences Division, Subscription Customer Service, 3251 Riverport Lane, Maryland Heights, MO 63043. **Customer Service: 1-800-654-2452 (U.S. and Canada); 314-447-8871 (outside U.S. and Canada). Fax: 314-447-8029. E-mail: journalscustomerservice-usa@elsevier.com (for print support); journalsonlinesupport-usa@elsevier.com (for online support).**

Reprints. For copies of 100 or more, of articles in this publication, please contact the Commercial Reprints Department, Elsevier Inc., 360 Park Avenue South, New York, NY 10010-1710. Tel. 212-633-3874; Fax: 212-633-3820; E-mail: reprints@elsevier.com.

Primary Care: Clinics in Office Practice is covered in *MEDLINE/PubMed (Index Medicus) and EMBASE/Excerpta Medica, Current Contents/Clinical Medicine, and ISI/BIOMED.*

Contributors

CONSULTING EDITOR

JOEL J. HEIDELBAUGH, MD, FAAFP, FACG
Clinical Professor, Departments of Family Medicine and Urology, Director of Medical Student Education and Clerkship Director, Department of Family Medicine, University of Michigan Medical School, Ann Arbor, Michigan, USA; Ypsilanti Health Center, Ypsilanti, Michigan, USA

EDITORS

VINCENT MORELLI, MD
Professor, Department of Family and Community Medicine, Meharry Medical College, Professor Adjunct, Vanderbilt University, Nashville, Tennessee, USA

JOEL J. HEIDELBAUGH, MD, FAAFP, FACG
Clinical Professor, Departments of Family Medicine and Urology, Director of Medical Student Education and Clerkship Director, Department of Family Medicine, University of Michigan Medical School, Ann Arbor, Michigan, USA; Ypsilanti Health Center, Ypsilanti, Michigan, USA

AUTHORS

DUNCAN Y. AMEGBLETOR, PhD
Data Scientist, Department of Psychiatry and Behavioral Sciences, Meharry Medical College, Nashville, Tennessee, USA

VANISHA BROWN, PhD, MPH
Assistant Professor, School of Graduate Studies, Meharry Medical College, Nashville, Tennessee, USA

NICHOLAS CONLEY, MD
Medical Director, Cooperative Recovery, Medical Director, Integrated Health Cooperative at Mental Health Cooperative, Nashville, Tennessee, USA

MEKEILA C. COOK, MS, PhD
Assistant Professor, Division of Public Health Practice, School of Graduate Studies and Research, Meharry Medical College, Nashville, Tennessee, USA

GREEN EKADI, PhD
Professor, School of Graduate Studies, Meharry Medical College, Nashville, Tennessee, USA

CHRISTOPHER J. FRANK, MD, PhD
Clinical Assistant Professor, Department of Family Medicine, University of Michigan, Ann Arbor, Michigan, USA

DANNY GOLDBERG, MA
Research Director, Grow2Learn Cooperative, Madison, Tennessee, USA

SANDRA J. GONZALEZ, PhD, MSSW
Assistant Professor, Department of Family and Community Medicine, Baylor College of Medicine, Houston, Texas, USA

RACHEL HANEBUTT, EdM, MA
Doctoral Student in the Community Research and Action Program, Department of Human and Organizational Development, Vanderbilt University Peabody College, Nashville, Tennessee, USA

MARIE HANNA, MD
Resident, PGY-3, Department of Family Medicine, Meharry Medical College, Nashville, Tennessee, USA

BRYAN W. HECKMAN, PhD
Associate Professor, Department of Psychiatry and Behavioral Sciences, Economic Development University Center Director, Division of Public Health, School of Graduate Studies and Research, Meharry Medical College, Nashville, Tennessee, USA

ROBERT JOSEPH HEIZELMAN, MD
Clinical Instructor, Department of Family Medicine, Director, Medical Informatics, University of Michigan, Ann Arbor, Michigan, USA

JACQUELINE M. HIRTH, PhD, MPH
Assistant Professor, Department of Family and Community Medicine, Baylor College of Medicine, Houston, Texas, USA

PAUL D. JUAREZ, PhD
Professor and Vice Chair for Research, Department of Family and Community Medicine, Meharry Medical College, Nashville, Tennessee, USA

MEREDITH L. MEADOWS, MS
Doctoral Student in Community, Research and Action, Department of Human and Organizational Development, Vanderbilt University, Nashville, Tennessee, USA

HASINA MOHYUDDIN, PhD
Assistant Dean, Peabody Office of Equity, Diversity and Inclusion, Research Associate and Lecturer, Department of Human and Organizational Development, Vanderbilt University Peabody College, Nashville, Tennessee, USA

VINCENT MORELLI, MD
Professor, Department of Family and Community Medicine, Meharry Medical College, Professor Adjunct, Vanderbilt University, Nashville, Tennessee, USA

LEIGH MORRISON, MD
Clinical Assistant Professor, Department of Family Medicine, University of Michigan, Ann Arbor, Michigan, USA

JAMES MUCHIRA, PhD, RN
Assistant Professor, Vanderbilt University School of Nursing, Nashville, Tennessee, USA

JOHN K. MUTHUKA, PhD
Faculty of Public Health /Research, Kenya Medical Training College, Nairobi, Kenya

ROSEMARY NABAWEESI, MBChB, DrPH
RWJF Endowed Chair for Health Policy, Associate Professor, Center for Health Policy, School of Graduate Studies, Meharry Medical College, Nashville, Tennessee, USA

HEATHER M. O'HARA, MD, MPH
Associate Professor, Department of Family and Community Medicine, Meharry Medical College, Medical Director, Memorial Occupational Health Clinic, Decatur, Illinois, USA

DEREK A. POPE, PhD
Adjunct Faculty, Department of Psychiatry and Behavioral Sciences, Meharry Medical College, Nashville, Tennessee, USA

COLEMAN PRATT, MD
Assistant Professor, Department of Family and Community Medicine, Tulane University School of Medicine, New Orleans, Louisiana, USA

ADRIAN D. SAMUELS, PhD
Senior Vice President for Student Affairs, Executive Director, Center for Health Policy, School of Graduate Studies, Meharry Medical College, Nashville, Tennessee, USA

DAWN SCHWARTZ, MEd
Project Manager, Department of Health Policy, Vanderbilt University Medical Center, Nashville, Tennessee, USA

STACY D. SMITH, MD
Resident, PGY-2, Department of Family and Community Medicine, Meharry Medical College, Nashville, Tennessee, USA

RUTH STEWART, MD
Associate Dean of Medical Education, Departments of Family and Community Medicine, and Professional and Medical Education, Meharry Medical School, Nashville, Tennessee, USA

SARAH V. SUITER, PhD, MS
Associate Professor in Human and Organizational Development, Vanderbilt University, Nashville, Tennessee, USA

RILEY TAYLOR, MD, MPH
Fellow Physician, Department of Preventive Medicine, Cook County Health, Chicago, Illinois, USA

CAROL ZIEGLER, DNP, APRN, NP-C, APHN-BC
Professor, Vanderbilt University School of Nursing, Nashville, Tennessee, USA

ROGER ZOOROB, MD, MPH, FAAFP
Richard M. Kleberg, Sr. Professor and Chair, Department of Family and Community Medicine, Baylor College of Medicine, Houston, Texas, USA

Contents

Foreword: The Meaning Behind the Medicine xiii

Joel J. Heidelbaugh

Preface: Twenty-First Century Challenge: Social Determinants of Health xv

Vincent Morelli and Joel J. Heidelbaugh

PART ONE: SOCIAL DETERMINANTS AS DEFINED BY THE CDC

Social Determinants of Health: An Overview for the Primary Care Provider 507

Vincent Morelli

Social determinants of health (SDoH) are reflected in how people live (access to health care, economic stability, built environment, food security, climate), learn (the educational environment), work (occupational environment), and play/socialize (social context and digital domain). All of these day-to-day conditions play a vital role in a patient's overall health, and a primary care provider should be prepared to understand their role to screen, assess, and address SDoH in clinical practice.

Monitoring Social Determinants of Health Assessing Patients and Communities 527

Vincent Morelli and Robert Joseph Heizelman

Because of the devastating health effects of social determinants of health (SDoH), it is important for the primary care provider to assess and monitor these types of stressors. This can be done via surveys, geomapping, or various biomarkers. To date, however, each of these methods is fraught with obstacles. There are currently are no validated "best" SDoH screening tools for use in clinical practice. Nor is geomapping, a perfect solution. Although mapping can collect location specific factors, it does not account for the fact that patients may live in one area, work in another and travel frequently to a third.

Health Equity and Access to Health Care as a Social Determinant of Health: The Role of the Primary Care Provider 549

Coleman Pratt, Riley Taylor, and Stacy D. Smith

Populations of people who suffer poorer health outcomes and increased disease burden, particularly preventable diseases, injury, and violence are experiencing health inequity. Achieving greater health equity by addressing social determinants of health and access to health care is the goal of many primary care physicians, health care advocates, and policy makers. Race, geographic location, age, poverty, disabilities, gender, and mental health are common examples of factors that determine health equity. Access to health care, by itself is a predictor of health outcomes and is influenced by many of the same factors.

Economic Determinants of Health Disparities and the Role of the Primary Care Provider 561

Paul D. Juarez

The economic determinants of adverse personal health outcomes and population level disparities pose a daunting challenge for primary care providers in promoting health for persons experiencing poverty and neighborhood deprivation. Until they are addressed, however, the health and economic well-being of persons experiencing neighborhood deprivation is not likely to be improved. There is growing evidence of effective interventions that primary care providers can adopt to address social and economic determinants of health. Primary care providers can participate in clinic and community-based approaches that target individual, neighborhood and social level drives of health and disparities.

Educational Attainment and Educational Contexts as Social Determinants of Health 579

Sarah V. Suiter and Meredith L. Meadows

Research demonstrates that nearly all health outcomes are patterned by level of education. Specifically, adults with lower educational attainment report more chronic conditions, more functional limitations, and worse overall health. In addition to affecting educational attainment, schools provide an important context in which students spend a substantial portion of their time. Because access to salutogenic school environments, as well as opportunities for educational attainment and advancement are themselves unequal, education is considered a social determinant of health. In this article, we explore the relationships between educational attainment and health. We also emphasize the importance of educational contexts as determinants of health that precede educational attainment and contribute to related health outcomes. Finally, we discuss implications for primary care practitioners and their efforts to address disparities in health and education.

The Built Environment as a Social Determinant of Health 591

Rosemary Nabaweesi, Marie Hanna, John K. Muthuka, Adrian D. Samuels, Vanisha Brown, Dawn Schwartz, and Green Ekadi

The built environment encompasses buildings we live in; the distribution systems that provide us with water and electricity; and the roads, bridges, and transportation systems we use to get from place to place. It provides safety, health, and well-being and meaning to its dwellers, as a place to work, live, learn, play, and thrive. Poor-quality housing affects dwellers' health through toxins such as radon and lead, mold, cold indoor temperatures, and overcrowding. Physicians' practices should investigate their patients' diagnoses such as stress, depression, asthma, adverse childhood experiences, and anxiety, as potentially housing-related and make ameliorating recommendations or referrals.

The Social Context: Social and Behavioral Factors That Affect Health Outcomes 601

Jacqueline M. Hirth, Sandra J. Gonzalez, and Roger Zoorob

To achieve understanding and best care, screening and treating patients should consider the patient's social environment. Social and behavioral factors influence both positive and negative health behaviors that influence mental and physical health. Primary care providers continually navigate barriers faced by patients and seek solutions that take into consideration social and behavioral factors. The role of the PCP begins with an understanding of common barriers and community resources, then by assessing and responding to the patient's own challenges, and finally by advocating in the clinic and public for changes to the underlying social and structural causes of morbidity and mortality.

The Work, Play, and Worship Environments as Social Determinants of Health **621**

Heather M. O'Hara

Consideration of the definition of the social determinants of health (SDOHs) requires health care to include work, play, and worship environments because they are important to the health of patients and communities. This article attempts to discuss the issues with limited focus on these areas and the importance of using multidisciplinary health-care teams during primary care visits. The expectation from this information is to advance the ability for primary care providers to support patients and the communities they work in to effect change toward decreasing health disparities and enhancing overall health outcomes.

Food and Nutrition Security as Social Determinants of Health: Fostering Collective Impact to Build Equity **633**

Duncan Y. Amegbletor, Danny Goldberg, Derek A. Pope, and Bryan W. Heckman

An overview of the state of the American diet, how it relates to public health outcomes and the obesity epidemic, and how it arises from the policy and infrastructure that have been developed over the course of the 20th and 21st centuries. The article concludes by laying out concrete solutions for urban revitalization, providing people in underserved communities sovereignty over their food supply, and work with multi-stakeholder cooperatives to overcome the effects of food insecurity and poor diet quality.

Climate Change: The Ultimate Determinant of Health **645**

Carol Ziegler and James Muchira

Climate change ubiquitously influences social determinants of health via various pathways. Disproportionately burdening communities who have contributed the least to greenhouse gas (GHG) emissions and benefitted the least from economic benefits obtained through high-emission activities that cause climate change, climate justice must be centered in any discussion of health equity. This article will explore how climate change contributes to health disparities in vulnerable populations, why this is a justice issue for primary care to address, and what we can do to promote equity, resilience, and adaption in our current economic system while mitigating GHG emissions, leveraging the health sector.

at the community level. The aftermath of the COVID-19 pandemic further highlighted the necessity for organizational resilience in the United States. The US public health and health care system began the lengthy process of identifying the resiliency needs of its workforce that expand beyond disaster preparedness. The purpose of this article is to describe the relationship between resilience and SDOH and how medical training can infuse resiliency within the curriculum and clinical practice.

PRIMARY CARE: CLINICS IN OFFICE PRACTICE

FORTHCOMING ISSUES

March 2024
Cardiovascular Diseases
Anthony Viera, *Editor*

June 2024
Neurology
Kara Wyant and Melissa Elafros, *Editors*

September 2024
Endocrinology
Michael Malone and Vasudha Jain, *Editors*

RECENT ISSUES

September 2023
Gastroenterology
Parvathi Perumareddi, *Editor*

June 2023
Allergy and Immunology
Andrew Lutzkanin III and Kristen M. Lutzkanin, *Editors*

March 2023
Behavioral Health
Meagan Vermeulen, *Editor*

Foreword
The Meaning Behind the Medicine

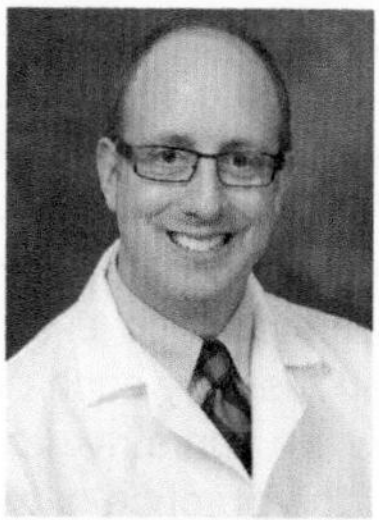

Joel J. Heidelbaugh, MD, FAAFP, FACG
Consulting Editor

As the landscape of medicine continues to rapidly evolve, and as we have rightfully recognized the importance of incorporating a greater scale of public health education in medical schools and residency programs, there remains a substantial need to provide continuing education on the impact of social determinants of health in primary care. This includes ongoing education and integration of key terms and concepts for health care providers in all facets of medicine and at all stages of their careers. When a proposal came forward to develop a singular issue of *Primary Care: Clinics in Office Practice* dedicated to social determinants of health that would detail over a dozen salient elements composed by an expert panel of scholars and authors, I immediately greenlit the project.

Several years ago, our medical students conducted a survey to ascertain both what we teach and what they learn with respect to the social determinants of health. The results were (embarrassingly) predictable: we weren't meeting their needs. What we also learned was that most faculty weren't equipped to teach the fundamentals. Admittedly many faculty defended that, "of course we do this stuff every day, with every patient," but conceded that there are greater depths of understanding that we must learn to better change the many disparities in health care if we are ever to improve outcomes in our communities.

This issue of *Primary Care: Clinics in Office Practice* is truly unique and is designed to be a blueprint for teaching aspects of social determinants of health across a wide spectrum of students, residents, and health care providers. The issue commences with a detailed overview and historical perspective for the primary care provider followed by information on how to assess and monitor social determinants through epigenetics, biomarkers, and regional mapping. Articles detail strategies to improve health equity through improving access to health care and economic stability, the learning environment, the built environment, the social context, and the work environment. Provocative articles highlight the roles of food insecurity, climate, and violence in

Prim Care Clin Office Pract 50 (2023) xiii–xiv
https://doi.org/10.1016/j.pop.2023.05.003
0095-4543/23/© 2023 Published by Elsevier Inc.

impacting social determinants throughout the life cycle. The issue ends with a very heartfelt article that tells the story of building resilience that I trust will inspire our readers. Having read this entire issue front to back several times, I have gained a new appreciation for what we might be doing on some level but have learned what we all need to be doing on a greater scale in patient advocacy and global education.

I am honored to work again with my long-time friend and collaborator, Dr Vincent Morelli, on this timely and important issue of *Primary Care: Clinics in Office Practice*. This project has been his brilliant vision and creation, which I know will have great impact in both the educational and the clinical arenas. I would also like to acknowledge the editing efforts and medical student perspective of Ms Kinsey Vear, who provided keen insight into strategies to augment both content and broad relevance of several articles. I offer my sincere gratitude to all of the authors and experts who crafted outstanding articles on the relevant subtopics herein, as they each provide a novel perspective on social determinants of health and how we can strive to change people's lives. For all of us, this is the true meaning behind the practice of medicine.

Joel J. Heidelbaugh, MD, FAAFP, FACG
Departments of Family Medicine and Urology
Department of Family Medicine
University of Michigan Medical School
Ann Arbor, MI, USA

Ypsilanti Health Center
200 Arnet Suite 200
Ypsilanti, MI 48198, USA

E-mail address:
jheidel@umich.edu

Preface

Twenty-First Century Challenge: Social Determinants of Health

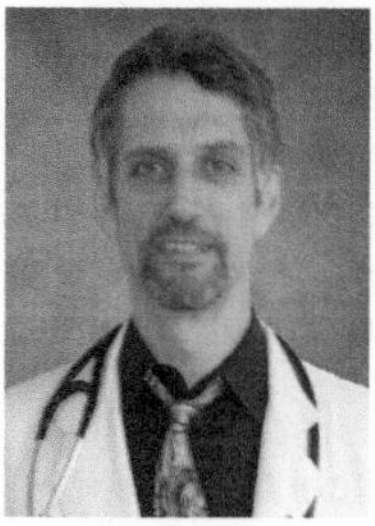

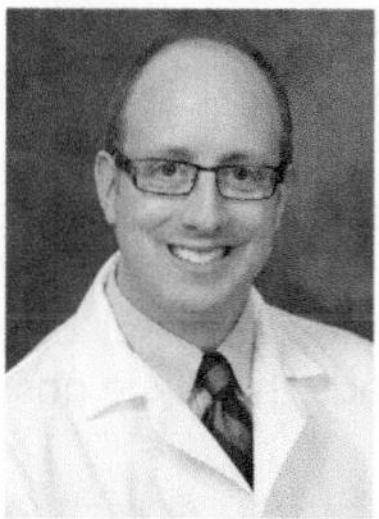

Vincent Morelli, MD Joel J. Heidelbaugh, MD, FAAFP, FACG
Editors

Public health efforts from the nineteenth century onward have made great strides in improving global health and longevity. Vaccines, food and water safety standards, occupational safety requirements, and educational campaigns focused on tobacco, drugs, and alcohol have all helped create a safer, healthier society. Clinical medicine, too, has contributed. The discovery of new drugs such as antibiotics and insulin, the implementation of antiseptic techniques and novel surgical methods, and the advancements in health care delivery systems all have played a role in converting what had previously been death sentences into routine, surmountable medical conditions. Today, in the twenty-first century, we face a different challenge: confronting the social determinants of health (SDoH). These nonmedical drivers of health outcomes, factors such as health care access, economic status, educational opportunity, built environments, social factors, workplace conditions, food security, and so forth, account for 40% of the modifiable health outcomes, while clinical intervention accounts for just 20%. This means that addressing SDoH in our patients is twice as important as addressing their presenting clinical issues in terms of long-term health. With this in mind, this issue reviews how SDoH impact physical and mental health, and will explore the role of the primary care provider (PCP) in ameliorating their effects. If we are to make the greatest impact on health outcomes in the twenty-first century, here is where we will have to focus our attention.

As PCPs, we are in a unique position to witness the effects of SDoH—from chronic physical maladies, such as heart disease, obesity, and cancer, to mental health issues like depression and anxiety, to the behavioral health fallout in the guise of drug and alcohol abuse, risky behaviors, and criminality. All of this has been linked to SDoH, a kind of “disenfranchisement syndrome” implicit in the many stress-related ailments

Prim Care Clin Office Pract 50 (2023) xv–xvi
https://doi.org/10.1016/j.pop.2023.05.001
0095-4543/23/© 2023 Published by Elsevier Inc.

that so often stunt the potential of our youth and slow the progression of our collective future.

As PCPs, we are best situated to screen, intervene, educate, and refer and, when possible, to use our "lived clinical experience" to help advocate for policy change. We are stationed between patients, public health, and policymakers with an important voice and a need to be at the table. We hope that primary care providers, medical educators, and policymakers will take the time to consider the information contained in this issue, whether in the clinical setting, in the medical classroom, or in the halls of government where future health care policies are set.

We are thankful to Meharry Medical College for allowing the time to complete this project and we are honored to have worked with such an accomplished group of author-collaborators, with Dr Joel Heidelbaugh, our long-time friend, collaborator and co-editor, with Mandy Vincent, our project coordinator, with Michael Trombadore our manuscript reviewer, and the entire publishing team at Elsevier – all of whom have made invaluable contributions and have made this issue possible.

Vincent Morelli, MD
Department of Family and Community Medicine
Meharry Medical College
3rd Floor, Old Hospital Building
1005 Dr DB Todd Jr Boulevard
Nashville, TN 37208-3599, USA

Joel J. Heidelbaugh, MD, FAAFP, FACG
Departments of Family Medicine and Urology
Department of Family Medicine
University of Michigan Medical School
Ann Arbor, MI, USA

Ypsilanti Health Center
200 Arnet Suite 200
Ypsilanti, MI 48198, USA

E-mail addresses:
morellivincent@gmail.com (V. Morelli)
jheidel@umich.edu (J.J. Heidelbaugh)

PART ONE: SOCIAL DETERMINANTS AS DEFINED BY THE CDC

Social Determinants of Health: An Overview for the Primary Care Provider

Vincent Morelli, MD

KEYWORDS

- Social determinants of health • Social risk factors • Economic stability
- Education access • Quality health care access • Quality neighborhood
- Built environment

KEY POINTS

- Addressing social determinants of health (SDoH) can be more impactful than clinical care.
- The constant stress of SDoH can overwhelm the body's immune responses.
- SDoH stresses impair the physical, mental, and behavioral health of the individual as well as health systems and communities.
- Most medical organizations advocate for incorporating SDoH screening in a health care visit, but there is no consensus on the best screening tools.
- Information about SDoH should be included in medical education.

INTRODUCTION

The World Health Organization (WHO) defines social determinants of health (SDoH) as, "non-medical factors that influence health outcomes. . . the conditions in which people are born, grow, work, live, and age, and the wider set of forces and systems shaping the conditions of daily life."[1] Such "forces and systems" include political and legal systems, social and economic policies, and societal and group norms—all man-made circumstances that shape the world's distribution of money, power, and resources, and all conditions that affect a wide range of health and quality-of-life risks and outcomes."[2]

In this volume of *Primary Care Clinics in Office Practice*, the author devotes manuscripts to the conditions in which people live (access to health care, economic stability, built environment, food security, climate as a social determinant), learn (educational environment), work (occupational environment), and play/socialize (social context

Department of Family & Community Medicine, Meharry Medical College, 3rd Floor, Old Hospital Building, 1005 Dr. D. B. Todd, Jr., Boulevard, Nashville, TN 37208-3599, USA
E-mail address: morellivincent@gmail.com

Prim Care Clin Office Pract 50 (2023) 507–525
https://doi.org/10.1016/j.pop.2023.04.004

and digital domain). The volume also contains works looking at how primary care providers (PCPs) might encounter SDoH in clinical practice. The goal of this second section is to build on the foundation laid out earlier and offer the PCP a more practical, clinical lens through which to view and address SDoH. The final manuscript in this volume, dedicated to resilience, provides the PCP with insights on ways to overcome suboptimal SDoH in individual patients and lays a foundation from which policy makers may begin the uphill battle for systems change.

Keeping in mind that the audience for this work is very broad including medical students, primary care residents, practicing clinicians, medical educators, and public health workers and policy makers, the purpose of this overview is to (1) provide a brief overview of the history of SDoH; (2) enhance awareness and emphasize the importance of SDoH; (3) provide an approach to assessing and addressing SDoH in the primary care setting; (4) propose how SDoH might be more fully integrated into medical education; and (5) serve a resource to inform and assist policy makers.

The History of Social Determinants of Health as a Health-Related Construct

Social and societal factors have impacted human health since the dawn of civilization. As far back as 10,000 years ago, the agricultural revolution brought with it social conditions that drastically increased the incidence of interpersonal violence and disease.[3,4]

In more modern times, the rapid changes of the Industrial Revolution of the 1800s spawned poor working conditions, pollution, and poverty, again markedly increasing disease and human suffering. The health effects were so apparent that prominent physician Rudolf Virchow (the father of modern pathology) stated, "If medicine is to fulfill her great task, then she must enter the political and social life. Do we not always find the diseases of the populace traceable to defects in society?"[5,6] Thus, the foundations of social medicine were laid, and the scientific community began to explore the roots of disease, not just in the biological setting but in the social realm as well.

International awareness of SDoH took a leap forward following WWII when the newly convened WHO defined health as "a state of complete physical, mental and social well-being," stating that health was preeminently shaped by societal conditions. This stance led the WHO to write into its constitution a pledge to "work with national governments to promote the improvement of nutrition, housing, sanitation, recreation, economic and working conditions."

Despite this, however, the WHOs vision was not immediately implemented. Instead, the focus of public health shifted away from social determinants to one focused on technological breakthroughs. The change was due to at least two factors. First, about this time, several scientific breakthroughs produced an array of new antibiotics, vaccines, and other medicines, giving the impression that technology was the answer to the world's health problems. Second, political factors played a role. At the time, the Soviet Union and the United States were quarreling over whether or not to include Soviet satellite states as full voting members of the United Nations (UN). When the United States vetoed such inclusion, the Soviets briefly dropped out of the UN in protest. During their absence, the United States and allies, eschewing the word "social," pushed against the SDoH model and instead championed a more capitalistic/technologic model focused on "curing" diseases.[7]

By the 1960s in the United States, a renewed interest in SDoH emerged when prevailing health systems were noted to do little to help poor and urban populations. In the 1970s, due, at least in part, to the drop in US prestige after the failures of the Vietnam War, the trend toward community-based health with a renewed focus on SDoH continued.[8–10]

Later, in 1978, a WHO-sponsored International Conference on Primary Health Care championed a primary health care (PHC) model involving health care systems and "all related sectors—including agriculture, animal husbandry, food, industry, education, housing, public works, and communication." The conference, attended by 3000 delegates from 134 governments, condemned global inequality and called for program "development in the spirit of social justice."

The successful (as measured by life expectancy and child mortality) rollout of this original PHC model was seen in China, Costa Rica, and Sri Lanka. The demonstrated effectiveness was attributed to five factors: a commitment to health as a social goal; a social welfare orientation to development; community participation in decision-making processes relative to health; and universal coverage of health services for all social groups (equity) and the intersectionality of health-related factors.[11] This latter element—intersectionality was judged most important as, for example, without food security and women's health literacy, universal health coverage or community involvement in decision making makes little difference.

Despite the above noted successes of the *original* PHC model, those committed to market-based health care were opposed to it. They believed that this broad "too idealistic" approach, which attempted to strengthen *all* aspects of health systems and to transform social and political systems simultaneously, was impractical.[12] Instead, they favored a *selective* PHC model which advocated a more pragmatic approach, emphasizing technical interventions and measurable outcomes.[13]

This *selective* PHC approach was swiftly adopted by influential global actors including the United States, The International Monetary Fund, and the World Bank. Thus, by the 1980s, with societal norms embracing the neoliberal vision, the conviction that free markets are the most efficient, most cost-effective allocators of resources,[14] the *selective* PHC model took hold. The ensuing years saw this neoliberal (meaning "less-government involvement") formula fail in Latin America and Asia, where the reforms proved unable to fulfill the stated goals of improving health outcomes or health equity and instead created greater inequity, more dissatisfaction, and lower economic efficiency.[15] A 2001 study concluded such programs were "inappropriately designed for developing country contexts" and were "quite out of touch with the reality of health systems and the broader socio-political environment."[16]

Today, the pendulum has begun to swing back toward the health-care-for-all paradigm with a renewed emphasis on SDoH.[17] Sweden, an early advocate to this paradigm, approved a public health strategy in 2002 that incorporated SDoH and was intent on creating, "societal conditions to ensure good health, on equal terms, for the entire population."[18] The trend was reinforced when Lee Jong-Wook, the newly elected WHO Director-General, launched the Commission on Social Determinants of Health in 2004. The commission was tasked with advancing equity and supporting countries—especially developing countries—with technical and policy support. Thus, via this tortuous path, we end up with the health-for-all-model back in favor on both the national and international stages.[19] It is clear that *now* is the time to capitalize on the zeitgeist to increase awareness of SDoH and make impactful and lasting changes.

Enhancing Primary Care Provider Awareness of the Importance of Social Determinants of Health

Research shows that public health measures addressing social determinants can be much more impactful than clinical care in influencing health outcomes. In fact, clinical intervention is said to be responsible for just 20% of modifiable health outcomes, whereas social determinants are responsible for 40%, the remaining 40% being attributable to public health measures.[20,21] This asymmetry holds true in terms of mortality as well, with medical care responsible for eliminating just 10% to 15% of preventable deaths,[20] whereas up to 72% of deaths are attributable to social determinants such as income, education, and employment,[22]with the number of deaths resulting from low education roughly equivalent to those resulting from myocardial infarction; the number of deaths due to racial segregation comparable to deaths from cerebrovascular disease; and deaths stemming from low social support being equal in magnitude to those caused by lung cancer.[23]

Mechanism: how social determinants of health exert their effects

In a word—stress, the constant wear and tear of suboptimal SDoH is believed to cause their downstream impacts. Ever-present poverty, low occupational status, or lack of social connectivity, for example, can eventually overcome the body's adaptive mechanisms and exact a crushing toll on individual health.[24] Indeed, stress-related cortisol dysregulation, neurologic effects, developmental alterations, cellular adjustments, and epigenetic changes have all been associated with SDoH and linked to overall negative impacts in health outcomes, morbidity, and mortality.[25]

Such stress not only affects the life of the individual but can also be felt across generations—with stress leading to epigenetic changes and altered gene expression that can be passed on to future generations (eg, a poor diet in parents or grandparents can influence trends toward obesity in offspring).[26] In essence, disadvantaged parents who are adversely affected by SDoH can pass on greater morbidity and mortality to their children.[27]

The fallout from suboptimal social determinants of health

Although the fallout from social determinants in many cases is obvious (who doesn't know that high-crime neighborhoods can lead to higher mortality or that low social connectivity to depression?), a closer look will heighten awareness of the degree of impact and intersectionality.

Biological impact. Psychological stress induces a number of physiologic actions including activation of the hypothalamic–pituitary axis and the sympathetic nervous system, elevating cortisol and catecholamine levels and activating their downstream receptors.[28,29] Of particular importance here is the effect that stress has on the developing brain-documented neurologic delays and deficits in the amygdala, hippocampus, prefrontal cortex, and mesolimbic reward circuits.[30–32] These insults create measurable neuro-structural changes that in turn can affect learning, cause behavioral and mental health issues, and result in the risky behaviors that affect both individuals and communities.

On a cellular level, suboptimal SDoH have also been associated with epigenetic changes,[33] telomere degradation,[34,35] as well as changes in other biomarkers.[36–38] These are discussed in depth in the next chapter.

Physical health impact. SDoH are strongly implicated in the physical health inequalities seen in disadvantaged populations throughout the world. Disenfranchised individuals are subject to higher child mortality, greater incidence of disease throughout life, and lower life expectancy.[39]

For example, the two leading causes of death in developed countries, cardiovascular disease and cancer, are strongly associated with SDoH. A 2020 study published in *Lancet* found that metabolic factors (eg, lipids, blood pressure, diabetes, obesity, tobacco, alcohol, diet, exercise, and salt) —all factors greatly influenced by SDoH—accounted for 41% of cardiovascular (CV) *events* (eg, myocardial infarction [MI], congestive heart failure [CHF], CVA), with air pollution alone responsible for 14%. The study went on to document that SDoH were responsible for 26% of cardiovascular *deaths* and, perhaps surprisingly, that low education was the biggest single causative SDoH, accounting for 13% of deaths by itself.[40] Such striking findings have prompted the American Heart Association to issue their Scientific Statement on Social Determinants of Health, declaring "Although we have traditionally considered CVD the consequence of modifiable (lifestyle) and nonmodifiable (genetic) risk factors, we must now broaden the focus to incorporate a third arm of risk: the social determinants of health. The most significant opportunities for reducing death and disability from CVD in the US lie with addressing the social determinants of cardiovascular outcomes."[41]

In terms of the second leading cause of death in the United States, cancer and social determinants are similarly linked. SDoH is associated with lower levels of colon cancer screening, a higher incidence of disease, and worse surgical outcomes.[42,43] Breast, lung, and prostate cancer are also linked to SDoH. In each case, SDoH have been associated with later diagnoses, more aggressive cancers, and poorer survival, with poverty, lack of education, lack of social support, and social isolation all playing a role.[44]

In terms of all-cause mortality and non-cancer–non-cardiovascular mortality, both are clearly increased in those with suboptimal SDoH. In a rigorous study examining lower socioeconomic and occupational status (eg, the social context and the work environment),[22] the investigators first confirmed earlier studies documenting the strong association of status with unhealthful behaviors such as increased smoking, unhealthy diet, and low levels of physical activity,[45,46] then went on to substantiate that increased mortality was associated with these behaviors over time (24 years in the cited study). The investigators found that these behaviors accounted for 72% of the disparity in all-cause mortality; 45% of the disparity in cardiovascular mortality; and 94% of the disparity in non-cancer–non-cardiovascular (eg, diabetes, liver disease, chronic obstructive pulmonary disease [COPD]) mortality.

Mental health impact. Turning briefly to mental and behavioral health, unemployment and stressful employment have been clearly linked with psychological distress and poor mental health,[47,48] as have lower income and financial strain.[49,50] Similarly, housing issues, neighborhood safety and food security, discrimination, social support, family relations, and immigration status have all been linked to anxiety, depression, and other mental health issues in a variety of countries.[48,50–52]

In addition to the toll that detrimental SDoH can have on most people's mental health, one must also consider patients with baseline mental health diagnoses. Such patients will experience (or already have experienced) a cyclical amplification of unhealthful fallout, with mental health issues leading to a deterioration of SDoH (eg, housing, social connection), leading to exacerbations of mental health issues, leading to further degradation of SDoH, leading to cumulating, cyclical harm.[53,54]

Behavioral health impact. Behavioral impacts such as smoking, substance use,[55] poor nutritional choices, and failing to exercise are clear downstream behavioral manifestations associated with SDoH.[55–57] Alcohol abuse is also a documented behavioral consequence of suboptimal SDoH. Neighborhoods with a high concentration of liquor stores result in a "behavioral nudge" and a resultant higher abuse of alcohol.[58] Similarly, crime, violent crime, and antisocial behaviors can be behavioral presentations of substandard SDoH. Economic instability, unsafe violent neighborhoods, and low educational attainment are all associated determinants both in the United States and internationally.[59–61]

Health system impact. SDoH and the associated physical, behavioral, and mental fallout seen in individual patients can combine in ways to create a substantial health system impact. For example, SDoH-causing mental health conditions can lead to medical nonadherence and inadequate self-care. This worsens both the psychologic condition itself and any concomitant physical conditions requiring adherence—all this compounded by the difficulty such a patient might have navigating through the health care system. The compounding effects of SDoH on physical, mental, and behavioral health, combined with their impact on noncompliance and delay of care can sabotage health efforts and dramatically increase health system costs.[62,63]

We can speculate about other hidden costs of SDoH by examining the diagnoses of simple office visits. For example, looking at the 72 million orthopedic office visits in the United States in 2018, one wonders how frequently SDoH might have played a role in presenting complaints such as low back pain or degenerative rotator cuff tendinopathy. Living in an unsafe neighborhood or with economic instability can dissuade exercise, eventually leading to degenerative tendinopathies, employment or disability issues, to further economic instability, and depression in a cyclical vortex. Similar invisible impacts of SDoH may be easily imagined when examining the 70 million annual cardiovascular office visits or the 60 million annual pulmonary visits.

Despite the much-discussed effect of SDoH on health system costs, we could find no clear estimate of the overall financial burden imposed by SDoH. This is likely due to the complex nature of their interactions—both between individual determinants and determinants and underlying medical conditions.[64] However, we can get an idea of the scope of the cost involved if we look at just one consequence of suboptimal SDoH: nonadherence. This is an issue proven to be associated with the determinants of poverty, social isolation, food insecurity, housing instability, and inadequate transportation.[65–70] This, coupled with the fact that half of US adults have at least one chronic medical condition,[71] has led researchers to estimate that the annual cost of medication noncompliance in the United States in 2018 to be between $495 and $673 billion—over 16% of US total annual health care expenditures.[72]

In terms of *appointment* compliance, as many as 20% to 30% of patients fail to keep their appointments, with a total estimated annual health system cost in 2010 to be over $150 billion/year[68,73,74] (we could find no more recent estimates). Although the literature has not, as yet, teased out how much noncompliance can be attributed to SDoH alone,[75] it is likely to be a substantial portion.

In sum, although the costs are difficult to estimate, the health system impacts of SDoH are substantial and some alternative payment models (eg, capitation, accountable care organizations) are beginning to consider SDoH and population health as a means of reducing utilization and cutting costs, most health systems have yet to fully embrace the use of social, mental, and behavioral services. They are just beginning to realize the complexity involved and the cyclical amplification of the effects of SDoH.[64]

Societal impact. The physical, mental, and behavioral issues afflicting a nation's denizens are costly to societies, burdening them with high educational-dropout rates, disability rates, incarceration rates, homelessness, and burdening them with indirect costs such as lost earnings, lower worker motivation, and lost productivity. Such issues make estimating full societal costs difficult. Despite this, due to the crippling effect that SDoH can have on individual citizens, a country's economy and its sense of civic well-being, it seems prudent to invest more heavily in the full physical, mental, and emotional development of citizens by accounting for SDoH in national policy.

Such an approach promises benefits for individuals, families, communities, and societies.[76]

A Primary Care Provider Approach to Assessing and Addressing Social Determinants of Health

Screening for social determinants of health: the role of the primary care provider

Recognizing the importance of SDoH, multiple organizations, including the American Academy of Pediatrics (AAP), the American Academy of Family Physicians (AAFP), and the American College of Physicians, have all endorsed screening and intervention.[77–80] Despite this philosophical concordance, and despite the fact that many organizations are doing "something" in this regard, most have yet to arrive at an agreed on the list of SDoH and, as a result, are often not fully aligned in their efforts to address them. For example, child maltreatment, childcare, child education, family financial support, physical environment, family social support, intimate partner violence, maternal depression, family mental illness, household substance abuse, firearm exposure, and parental health literacy are all seen as primary SDoH in pediatric spheres,[81] whereas other agencies list housing, transportation, and the safety as more significant.[82]

In addition to the lack of consensus on a comprehensive list of social determinants, the psychometric validity of screening tools has not yet been established, nor is there clear evidence regarding the efficacy of intervention and prevention programs. Nor is it known which SDoH might have greater impacts on which outcomes, which should be prioritized, or if certain clusters of determinants are especially damaging. For example, we are not sure if we should address housing before economics or how effective intervening with education is when we fail to provide economic stability and housing.

PCPs may also have ethical hesitations, questioning whether it is appropriate to screen and create expectations in disenfranchised populations if they cannot guarantee effective evidence-based interventions.[83] Cultural barriers, too, must be considered and many providers may not feel adequately trained to approach all patients in our multicultural society. For example, female Muslim patients may not be comfortable answering questions asked by male providers, or racially or economically disenfranchised populations may perceive SDoH questions to be intrusive or prejudicial.

As stated, despite these barriers and shortcomings[84,85] most medical organizations still advocate for incorporating SDoH screening into health care visits, noting that this should be done within the established guidelines of the U.S. Preventive Services Task Force (USPSTF) in the following manner: First, the targeted SDoH must be *individual* (eg, community-level determinants, such as community violence, or built environment inadequacy should not be addressed in this setting.) Second, the targeted determinant must be modifiable. Finally, screening, intervention, and referral should be initiated in the primary care setting where trusting relationships have already been established.[86]

However, in clinical medical practice, this is rarely done. Even attuned pediatric practices properly screen less than 25% of the time[87] and fewer still "close the loop" by following referrals and outcomes.[81,88,89] The reasons for this implementation gap, noted in roughly two-thirds of surveyed physicians, are lack of time, resources, training, knowledge, and/or compensation.[85,89]

Thus, as PCPs are largely unwilling, untrained, or unable to incorporate SDoH protocols into busy practices, there is a current trend toward a team-based approach to social determinant screening.[77,81]

In this team-based model, the PCPs role might include (1) choosing an age-appropriate written screening tool while accounting for the local cultural, racial, and economic conditions in his or her practice; (2) incorporating both risk and protective factors into the chosen screener; (3) training team members to administer the surveys using general, open-ended questions; (4) educating patients regarding the associated health effects and prioritizing intervention while considering patient and caregiver concerns; (4) documenting all this in the patient electronic medical record (EMR) and coding appropriately; and (5) facilitating referrals in a seamless manner.[81,83,90–92]

Currently, several such team-screening approaches are being evaluated. One of the most widely implemented protocols being beta-tested in 31 areas across the nation is the Accountable Health Communities (AHC) Model, supported by the Centers for Medicare and Medicaid Services. This team-administered survey examines five core domains: housing instability, food insecurity, transportation difficulties, utility assistance needs, and interpersonal safety and eight subdomains: financial status, employment, family and community support, education, physical activity, substance use, mental health, and disabilities.[82,93] The AHC model is a 5-year project, begun in 2018, which should soon begin publishing findings in terms of survey psychometric validity, patient acceptability, compliance and efficacy of referral, health outcomes, and cost analysis. The full 26-question AHC screening tool can be accessed at: https://innovation.cms.gov/files/worksheets/ahcm-screeningtool.

The AAFP also has a recommended screening tool: a 15-item survey that includes housing, food, transportation, utilities, education, finances, and safety which can be found at: https://www.aafp.org/dam/AAFP/documents/patient_care/everyone_project/hops19-physician-form-sdoh.pdf, and AAP has a myriad different screening tools available at https://www.aap.org/en/patient-care/screening-technical-assistance-and-resource-center/screening-resource-library/social-determinants-of-health/?page=1&sortDirection=1&sortField=Year.

Again, with none of the above tools yet validated, and none adequately considering the complexity, interconnected nature, or clustering effects that may be involved,[64,94,95] the PCP is left without definitive clinical guidance.

Still, some direction may be gained by looking at successful interventions that have been documented in studies examining *individual* determinants as discussed below. Although many of these are community-level interventions and are thus beyond the reach of the PCP, it is important that the PCP be aware of such successes to inform their own clinical interventions and to refer patients to appropriate community services.

Education

Early childhood education and social–emotional intervention has been shown to result in lower rates of risky behaviors (eg, smoking, drug use),[96] violent crime, incarceration, utilization of government assistance programs and higher educational attainment, income, and health insurance coverage—all this being manifested in adulthood some 40 years later.[97] Early education interventions have also resulted in lower rates of depression, more active lifestyles, lower body mass indices, and fewer risk factors for cardiovascular and metabolic disease.[98–100] Return-on-investment estimates for these and similar programs yield savings of 3 to 17 dollars per dollar invested,[101] translating to a roughly $18,000 cost reduction over the lifetime of each child enrolled.

Food

Food insecurity is a social determinant in 10% of US households, 90% of which are in the rural south. Such insecurity can result in higher smoking rates, less physical activity, type 2 diabetes mellitus, hypertension, cardiovascular disease,[102] psychological distress, poor sleep, depression, anxiety, and loneliness,[103,104] as well increased emergency department visits, inpatient admissions, and higher health care costs.[105]

Community-level coalition building and community input focused on policy change has been proven to help reduce food insecurity.[106] Other effective measures include income distribution, the elimination of food deserts (especially when teamed with educational programs), and the creation of "food pharmacies," the free food/produce distribution hubs staffed with dieticians to provide monthly educational programming and appropriate referral to other available community services.[105,107,108]

The built environment

Where people live is an especially impacting social determinant, with health outcomes significantly affected by neighborhood inequities[109] such as differences in chemical exposures, mold, pests, poor access to water or sanitation, proximity to pollution sources, lighting, green and recreational spaces, and so forth.[110] Thoughtful urban planning and interventions in housing stability, though outside of the realm of the PCP, can be a bulwark against these inequities and has been proven to positively affect dietary behaviors,[107] activity levels,[111] crime, violent crime, and drug and alcohol use,[58,61] employment, and social connectedness.[51,52,112,113] Other planning policies such as those advocating for placing primary care clinics in underserved neighborhoods rather than supporting remote specialty hospitals can offer additional individual and system-wide benefit.[114]

The workplace

The effects of an unstable work environment are significant, having been documented to adversely impact cardiovascular health and increased rates of myocardial infarction.[115] Conversely, reducing workplace discrimination has been shown to be of great benefit—a glaring example being the civil rights nondiscriminatory hiring policies instituted in the 1960s leading to income gains and increased life expectancy in just 10 years after implementation.[116]

Again, though out of the realm of PCP intervention, discussing the issue with patients may allow them to reframe the issue or take action to improve their situation.

Finances/economics

Several programs have been instituted in recent years providing citizens with basic universal income—foundational incomes, which were theorized to alleviate stress in under-resourced citizens and enable them to make better decisions, become healthier, and integrate more fully as productive members of society. Despite early indications of benefits, especially with programs such as social security (proven to lower mortality in the elderly) or American Indian youth supplement programs (demonstrating improved mental, behavioral and educational outcomes),[117,118] the most recent Cochrane review calls such benefits into question[119] stating, "The evidence on the relative effectiveness remains very uncertain." There are currently more nuanced and rigorous studies examining the concept currently underway in Kenya, the Netherlands, Uganda, Germany, and several US cities. Again, although beyond the interventional capacity of PCPs, knowledge of such programs may shift physician perception and allow for more meaningful patient interaction and effective referral.

The social environment

Improving social connectivity has been proven to impact health, beneficially affecting mental health outcomes in several studies. Programs that enhance youth engagement with school activities, adult or parental relationships, primary care relationships, and social media have all been linked to improvement in youth mental and behavioral health outcomes.[120] Similarly, effective interventions to combat social isolation in the elderly include involvement in face-to-face health and wellness programs, senior centers, faith-based organizations, and enhanced virtual connectivity.[121] Conversely, lack of social connection and loneliness has been said to carry the same health impact as smoking a half pack of cigarettes per day.[122] Here, as with other SDoH, the PCP may play a more active role in empathetic listening, patient education, intervention, and/or referral.

The above information is a brief overview of some of the effective SDoH interventions to date, all of which will be looked at in depth in subsequent chapters. For our purposes here though, the PCPs role of screening and addressing SDoH can be summarized as follows. It should include a team-based approach with a team member providing and encouraging the completion of an organizational screening tool (eg, AAFP, AAP), a subsequent PCP review with patients and caregivers, providing patient educating, recommencing intervention when appropriate, and having systems in place to arrange referrals, monitoring, and follow-up.

Integrating Social Determinants of Health into Medical Education

Medical educators have only recently begun to incorporate SDoH into medical school curricula, and educators are facing several challenges as they begin to do so. A 2019 review of SDoH in medical education[123] found that even in those schools where SDoH curriculum *did* exist, it was often taught by faculty with suboptimal experience and varying expertise, was conducted in the classroom setting, and was rarely performed in an inculcating longitudinal fashion. In addition, from a best teaching methods standpoint, there was variable incorporation of transformative or experiential learning. In agreement with studies cited above, the review noted that insufficient patient encounter time and lack of reimbursement were significant barriers to implementing SDoH into clinical teaching during third- and fourth-year clerkships.

As educators continue to initiate or strive to improve SDoH curricula, they may be helped by consulting models such as Kern's six-step curricula development model.[124] Such a paradigm focuses on transformative learning, involves service learning, and always includes critical reflection as an integral element. The goal of such a curriculum is to help make students: (1) more cognizant of social determinants and their associated health effects; (2) more skillful at screening and referral; (3) more adept at helping patients navigate through the health care system; and (4) ultimately, more capable in mitigating the health effects of SDoH.

Medical educators (including PCPs involved in clinical teaching), when designing such a curriculum should include the following components: (1) initial didactic sessions and reading assignments examining SDoH and their related health fallout; (2) visiting disadvantaged or immigrant communities through governmental agencies or NGOs whose missions addresses SDoH; (3) participating in case-based learning or neighborhood mapping exercises that incorporate SDoH; (4) working in disadvantaged family-centered clinics dealing with the physical, mental, or behavioral issues that result from SDoH; (5) participating in postexposure colloquium or group discussions; (5) completing surveys that create a space for critical reflection and the evaluation of learner experiences during the conclusion of longitudinal programming; and (6) for those especially moved by such experiences, elective credit might be given for creative engagement such as designing specific programs, apps, or games surrounding the issues.[125–129]

Critical reflection and transformational learning should be integral to designing any SDoH curriculum, as both have been proven to significantly impact learning, especially in regard to vulnerable populations and structural injustice.[130–132] (Definitions and discussions of transformative learning, service learning, and critical reflection in the context of medical education can be found in an excellent 2019 review by Doobay-Persaud and colleagues[123]).

When spelled out in this manner, the role of PCPs in such a curriculum becomes apparent. First, there is a responsibility to become educated themselves regarding SDoH. Then, it is important for them to participate in medical school didactic sessions and colloquiums bringing “lived experience” to the academic setting. Next PCPs should provide informed mentorship as students rotate through clinics during clinical clerkships, modeling best teaching methods in patient education interactions. Finally, it is incumbent on PCPs to discuss the importance of wrap-around services and follow-up as they provide referrals—discuss their particular referral panel and follow-up protocols thus demonstrating a more informed, whole-person, system's approach to rotating students. The implementation of medical curricula in a wide-spread fashion will not be easy, but it must be done if we are to impact the most pressing health issues of our day.

Providing a Resource to Inform Policy Makers

We hope that this volume will prove useful not only for PCPs, but also to the educators, public health researchers and policy makers who are just beginning to take note of the individual and societal costs associated with SDoH. Even though to date, studies evaluating interventions have met with mixed results,[133–135] and studies so far have proven unable to estimate the full costs associated with SDoH,[136] there is a pressing need to move forward.

SUMMARY

If we are to achieve the Healthy People 2030s goal of, “creating social, physical, and economic environments that promote attaining the full potential for health and well-being for all,” then we must work together toward intervening and improving the effects of suboptimal SDoH. There are roles for many players in this regard: public health workers, city planners, businesses, policy makers, politicians, and PCPs. Although it is clear that community and societal-level interventions are vital and clearly outside of the purview of clinicians, it is also clear that a PCP led team-based approach to screening and intervention is critical. Hopefully, this article has provided useful insights and a clearer perspective from which PCPs, researchers, community stakeholders, and lawmakers will be able to create more informed interventions, research projects, and policy in the future.

REFERENCES

1. World Health Organization. Social determinants of health. Available at: https://www.who.int/health-topics/social-determinants-of-health#tab=tab_1. Accessed January 20, 2023.
2. Centers for Disease Control and Prevention. Social Determinants of Health at CDC. Available at: https://www.cdc.gov/about/sdoh/index.html. Accessed January 01, 2023.
3. Diamond JM. Guns, germs, and steel: the fates of human societies. New York: W.W. Norton & Co.; 1997.
4. Walker RA, Bailey DH. Body counts in lowland South American violence. Evol Hum Behav 2013;34(1):29–34.
5. Szreter S. Industrialization and Health. Br Med Bull 2004;69:7586.

6. Lopez A, Caselli G, Valkonen T. In: *Adult mortality in developed countries: from description to explanation*. York: Oxford University Press; Oxford/New; 1995. p. 5–8.
7. Irwin A, Scali E. Action on the social determinants of health: a historical perspective. Glob Public Health 2007;2(3):235–56.
8. Cueto M. The origins of primary health care and selective primary health care. Am J Public Health 2004;94(11):1864–74.
9. Newell KW, WHO. Health by the people, 1975. Available at: https://apps.who.int/iris/handle/10665/40514. Accessed February 09, 2023.
10. Newell KW. Selective primary health care: the counter revolution. Soc Sci Med 1988;26(9):903–6.
11. Rosenfield P. The contribution of social and political factors to good health. In: Halstead S, Walsh J, Warren K, editors. Good health at low cost. New York: Rockefeller Foundation; 1985. 173-218.
12. Walsh JA, Warren KS. Selective primary health care: an interim strategy for disease control in developing countries. N Engl J Med 1979;301(18):967–74.
13. Brown TM, Cueto M, Fee E. The World Health Organization and the transition from "international" to "global" public health. Am J Public Health 2006;96(1): 62–72.
14. Coburn D. Income inequality, social cohesion and the health status of populations: the role of neo-liberalism. Soc Sci Med 2000;51(1):135–46.
15. Homedes N, Ugalde A. Why neoliberal health reforms have failed in Latin America. Health Pol 2005;71(1):83–96.
16. Mills A, Bennett S, Russell S. The challenge of health sector reform: what must governments do? Basingstoke: Palgrave; 2001.
17. Mackenbach J, Bakker M. In: *Reducing inequalities in health: a European perspective-*. London: Routledge; 2002. p. 26–8.
18. Swedish National Institute of Public Health. Sweden's new public health policy: national public health objectives for Sweden. Stockholm: National Institute of Public Health; 2003.
19. Lee JW. Speech to the 57th World Health Assembly, 18 May 2004. Available at: https://apps.who.int/iris/bitstream/handle/10665/20078/A57_3-en.pdf?sequence=1&isAllowed=y (Accessed February 02, 2023).
20. McGinnis JM, Williams-Russo P, Knickman JR. The case for more active policy attention to health promotion. Health Aff 2002;21(2):78–93.
21. Hood CM, Gennuso KP, Swain GR, et al. County health rankings: relationships between determinant factors and health outcomes. Am J Prev Med 2016;50: 129–35.
22. Stringhini S, Sabia S, Shipley M, et al. Association of Socioeconomic Position with Health Behaviors and Mortality. JAMA 2010;303:1159–66.
23. Galea S, Tracy M, Hoggatt KJ, et al. Estimated deaths attributable to social factors in the United States. Am J Pub Health 2011;101:1456–65.
24. Allen J, Balfour R, Bell R, et al. Social determinants of mental health. Int Rev Psych (Abingdon, England) 2014;26(4):392–407.
25. Johnson SB, Riis JL, Noble KG. State of the Art Review: Poverty and the Developing Brain. Pediatrics 2016;137(4):e20153075.
26. Daxinger L, Whitelaw E. Understanding transgenerational epigenetic inheritance via the gametes in mammals. Nat Rev Genet 2012;13(3):153–62.
27. Braveman P, Egerter S, Williams DR. The social determinants of health: coming of age. Annu Rev Public Health 2011;32:381–98.

28. Chrousos GP. Stress and disorders of the stress system. Nat Rev Endocrinol 2009;5(7):374–81.
29. Habib KE, Gold PW, Chrousos GP. Neuroendocrinology of stress. Endocrinol Metab Clin North Am 2001;30(3):695–viii.
30. Cook SC, Wellman CL. Chronic stress alters dendritic morphology in rat medial prefrontal cortex. J Neurobiol 2004;60(2):236–48.
31. Pervanidou P, Agorastos A, Chrousos GP. Editorial: Stress and Neurodevelopment. Front Neurosci 2022;16:898872.
32. Gold PW, Machado-Vieira R, Pavlatou MG. Clinical and biochemical manifestations of depression: relation to the neurobiology of stress. Neural Plast 2015;2015:581976.
33. Tung J, Barreiro LB, Johnson ZP, et al. Social environment is associated with gene regulatory variation in the rhesus macaque immune system. Proc Natl Acad Sci U S A 2012;109(17):6490–5.
34. Parks CG, Miller DB, McCanlies EC, et al. Telomere length, current perceived stress, and urinary stress hormones in women. Cancer Epidemiol Biomarkers Prev 2009;18(2):551–60.
35. Price LH, Kao HT, Burgers DE, et al. Telomeres and early-life stress: an overview. Biol Psychiatry 2013;73(1):15–23.
36. Lam PH, Chiang JJ, Chen E, et al. Race, socioeconomic status, and low-grade inflammatory biomarkers across the lifecourse: A pooled analysis of seven studies. Psychoneuroendocrinology 2021;123:104917.
37. Cozier YC, Albert MA, Castro-Webb N, et al. Neighborhood Socioeconomic Status in Relation to Serum Biomarkers in the Black Women's Health Study. J Urban Health 2016;93(2):279–91.
38. Singh-Manoux A, Shipley MJ, Bell JA, et al. Association between inflammatory biomarkers and all-cause, cardiovascular and cancer-related mortality. CMAJ (Can Med Assoc J) 2017;189(10):E384–90.
39. Alegría M, NeMoyer A, Falgàs Bagué I, et al. Social Determinants of Mental Health: Where We Are and Where We Need to Go. Curr Psychiatry Rep 2018;20(11):95.
40. Yusuf S, Joseph P, Rangarajan S, et al. Modifiable risk factors, cardiovascular disease, and mortality in 155 722 individuals from 21 high-income, middle-income, and low-income countries (PURE): a prospective cohort study. Lancet 2020;395(10226):795–808 [published correction appears in Lancet. 2020 Mar 7;395(10226):784].
41. Havranek EP, Mujahid MS, Barr DA, et al. Social Determinants of Risk and Outcomes for Cardiovascular Disease: A Scientific Statement From the American Heart Association. Circulation 2015;132(9):873–98.
42. Kane WJ, Fleming MA 2nd, Lynch KT, et al. Associations of Race, Ethnicity, and Social Determinants of Health with Colorectal Cancer Screening. Dis Colon Rectum 2022. https://doi.org/10.1097/DCR.0000000000002371 [published online ahead of print, 2022 May 9].
43. Pollak YLE, Lee JY, Khalid SI, et al. Social determinants of health Z-codes and postoperative outcomes after colorectal surgery: A national population-based study. Am J Surg 2022;224(5):1301–7.
44. Namburi N, Timsina L, Ninad N, et al. The impact of social determinants of health on management of stage I non-small cell lung cancer. Am J Surg 2022;223(6):1063–6.

45. Lynch JW, Kaplan GA, Salonen JT. Why do poor people behave poorly? Variation in adult health behaviours and psychosocial characteristics by stages of the socioeconomic lifecourse. Soc Sci Med 1997;44(6):809–19.
46. Martikainen P, Brunner E, Marmot M. Socioeconomic differences in dietary patterns among middle-aged men and women. Soc Sci Med 2003;56(7):1397–410.
47. Reibling N, Beckfield J, Huijts T, et al. Depressed during the depression: has the economic crisis affected mental health inequalities in Europe? Findings from the European Social Survey (2014) special module on the determinants of health. Eur J Public Health 2017;27(suppl_1):47–54.
48. Brydsten A, Hammarström A, San Sebastian M. Health inequalities between employed and unemployed in northern Sweden: a decomposition analysis of social determinants for mental health. Int J Equity Health 2018;17(1):59.
49. Amroussia N, Gustafsson PE, Mosquera PA. Explaining mental health inequalities in Northern Sweden: a decomposition analysis. Glob Health Action 2017;10(1):1305814.
50. Lecerof SS, Stafström M, Westerling R, et al. Does social capital protect mental health among migrants in Sweden? Health Promot Int 2016;31(3):644–52.
51. Han KM, Han C, Shin C, et al. Social capital, socioeconomic status, and depression in community-living elderly. J Psychiatr Res 2018;98:133–40.
52. Smyth N, Siriwardhana C, Hotopf M, et al. Social networks, social support and psychiatric symptoms: social determinants and associations within a multicultural community population. Soc Psychiatry Psychiatr Epidemiol 2015;50(7):1111–20.
53. Ljungqvist I, Topor A, Forssell H, et al. Money and Mental Illness: A Study of the Relationship Between Poverty and Serious Psychological Problems. Community Ment Health J 2016;52(7):842–50.
54. Hjorth CF, Bilgrav L, Frandsen LS, et al. Mental health and school dropout across educational levels and genders: a 4.8-year follow-up study. BMC Publ Health 2016;16:976.
55. Sugarman OK, Bachhuber MA, Wennerstrom A, et al. Interventions for incarcerated adults with opioid use disorder in the United States: A systematic review with a focus on social determinants of health. PLoS One 2020;15(1):e0227968.
56. Felitti VJ, Anda RF, Nordenberg D, et al. Relationship of childhood abuse and household dysfunction to many of the leading causes of death in adults. The Adverse Childhood Experiences (ACE) Study. Am J Prev Med 1998;14(4):245–58.
57. Dube SR, Anda RF, Felitti VJ, et al. Adverse childhood experiences and personal alcohol abuse as an adult. Addict Behav 2002;27(5):713–25.
58. LaVeist TA, Wallace JM Jr. Health risk and inequitable distribution of liquor stores in African American neighborhood. Soc Sci Med 2000;51(4):613–7.
59. Wanzinack C, Signorelli MC, Reis C. Violence and social determinants of health in Brazil: association between homicides, urbanization, population, inequality, and development. Cad Saúde Pública 2022;38(10):e00282621.
60. Blair KJ, de Virgilio M, Dissak-Delon FN, et al. Associations between social determinants of health and interpersonal violence-related injury in Cameroon: a cross-sectional study. BMJ Glob Health 2022;7(1):e007220.
61. Yu Q, Scribner R, Carlin B, et al. Multilevel spatio-temporal dual changepoint models for relating alcohol outlet destruction and changes in neighbourhood rates of assaultive violence. Geospat Health 2008;2(2):161–72.
62. Katon WJ, Lin EH, Von Korff M, et al. Collaborative care for patients with depression and chronic illnesses. N Engl J Med 2010;363(27):2611–20.

63. Morris RL, Sanders C, Kennedy AP, et al. Shifting priorities in multimorbidity: a longitudinal qualitative study of patient's prioritization of multiple conditions. Chronic Illn 2011;7(2):147–61.
64. Kuiper ME, Chambon M, de Bruijn AL, et al. A Network Approach to Compliance: A Complexity Science Understanding of How Rules Shape Behavior [published online ahead of print, 2022 May 10]. J Bus Ethics 2022;1–26. https://doi.org/10.1007/s10551-022-05128-8.
65. Wilder ME, Kulie P, Jensen C, et al. The Impact of Social Determinants of Health on Medication Adherence: a Systematic Review and Meta-analysis. J Gen Intern Med 2021;36(5):1359–70.
66. DiMatteo MR, Lepper HS, Croghan TW. Depression is a risk factor for noncompliance with medical treatment: meta-analysis of the effects of anxiety and depression on patient adherence. Arch Intern Med 2000;160(14):2101–7.
67. Wang M, Miller JD, Collins SM, et al. Social Support Mitigates Negative Impact of Food Insecurity on Antiretroviral Adherence Among Postpartum Women in Western Kenya. AIDS Behav 2020;24(10):2885–94.
68. Sviokla J, Schroede, B, Weakland T. How Behavioral Economics Can Help Cure the Health Care Crisis (March 1, 2010). Harvard Business Review 3;269:2779-2781. Available at: https://hbr.org/2010/03/how-behavioral-economics-can-h. (Accessed January 30, 23).
69. Peterson AM, Takiya L, Finley R. Meta-analysis of trials of interventions to improve medication adherence. Am J Health Syst Pharm 2003;60(7):657–65.
70. Haynes RB, Ackloo E, Sahota N, et al. Interventions for enhancing medication adherence. Cochrane Database Syst Rev 2008;2:CD000011.
71. Haynes RB, McDonald HP, Garg AX. Helping patients follow prescribed treatment: clinical applications. JAMA 2002;288(22):2880–3.
72. Watanabe JH, McInnis T, Hirsch JD. Cost of Prescription Drug-Related Morbidity and Mortality. Ann Pharmacother 2018;52(9):829–37.
73. Chariatte V, Berchtold A, Akré C, et al. Missed appointments in an outpatient clinic for adolescents, an approach to predict the risk of missing. J Adolesc Health 2008;43(1):38–45.
74. Triemstra JD, Lowery L. Prevalence, Predictors, and the Financial Impact of Missed Appointments in an Academic Adolescent Clinic. Cureus 2018;10(11):e3613.
75. Balkrishnan R. Predictors of medication adherence in the elderly. Clin Ther 1998;20(4):764–71.
76. National Academies of Sciences, Engineering, and Medicine; Division of Behavioral and Social Sciences and Education; Board on Children, Youth, and Families; Committee on Fostering Healthy Mental, Emotional, and Behavioral Development Among Children and Youth. Fostering Healthy Mental, Emotional, and Behavioral Development, In: *Children and youth: a national agenda*, 2019, National Academies Press (US), Washington, DC, 13-19.
77. O'Gurek DT, Henke C. A Practical Approach to Screening for Social Determinants of Health. Fam Pract Manag 2018;25(3):7–12.
78. Council on Community Pediatrics. Poverty and Child Health in the United States. Pediatrics 2016;137(4):e20160339.
79. Council on Community Pediatrics; Committee on Nutrition. Promoting Food Security for All Children. Pediatrics 2015;136(5):e1431–8.
80. Daniel H, Bornstein SS, Kane GC, et al. Addressing Social Determinants to Improve Patient Care and Promote Health Equity: An American College of Physicians Position Paper. Ann Intern Med 2018;168(8):577–8.

81. Chung EK, Siegel BS, Garg A, et al. Screening for Social Determinants of Health Among Children and Families Living in Poverty: A Guide for Clinicians. Curr Probl Pediatr Adolesc Health Care 2016;46(5):135–53.
82. Centers for Medicare & Medicaid Services. Accountable Health Communities Model. Available at: https://innovation.cms.gov/initiatives/ahcm. Accessed 06 January, 2023. (Accessed February 02, 2023).
83. Garg A, Boynton-Jarrett R, Dworkin PH. Avoiding the Unintended Consequences of Screening for Social Determinants of Health. JAMA 2016;316(8): 813–4.
84. Buitron de la Vega P, Losi S, Sprague Martinez L, et al. Implementing an EHR-based Screening and Referral System to Address Social Determinants of Health in Primary Care. Medical care 2019;57(Suppl 6 Suppl 2):S133–9.
85. Leavitt Partners. “Taking Action on Social Determinants of Health” Report, October 22, 2019. https://leavittpartners.com/press/leavitt-partners-releases-taking-action-on-social-determinants-of-health-report/. Accessed January 08, 2023.
86. Davidson KW, Kemper AR, Doubeni CA, et al. Developing Primary Care-Based Recommendations for Social Determinants of Health: Methods of the U.S. Preventive Services Task Force. Ann Intern Med 2020;173(6):461–7.
87. Friedman S, Caddle S, Motelow JE, et al. Improving Screening for Social Determinants of Health in a Pediatric Resident Clinic: A Quality Improvement Initiative. Pediatr Qual Saf 2021;6(4):e419.
88. Patel M, Bathory E, Scholnick J, et al. Resident Documentation of Social Determinants of Health: Effects of a Teaching Tool in the Outpatient Setting. Clin Pediatr (Phila) 2018;57(4):451–6.
89. Morgenlander MA, Tyrrell H, Garfunkel LC, et al. Screening for Social Determinants of Health in Pediatric Resident Continuity Clinic. Acad Pediatr 2019; 19(8):868–74.
90. Garg A, Butz AM, Dworkin PH, et al. Improving the management of family psychosocial problems at low-income children's well-child care visits: the WE CARE Project. Pediatrics 2007;120(3):547–58.
91. MacMillan HL, Wathen CN, Jamieson E, et al. Approaches to screening for intimate partner violence in health care settings: a randomized trial. JAMA 2006; 296(5):530–6.
92. Gottlieb L, Hessler D, Long D, et al. A randomized trial on screening for social determinants of health: the iScreen study. Pediatrics 2014;134(6):e1611–8.
93. Gottlieb L, Colvin JD, Fleegler E, et al. Evaluating the Accountable Health Communities Demonstration Project. J Gen Intern Med 2017;32(3):345–9.
94. Schiltz NK, Chagin K, Sehgal AR. Clustering of Social Determinants of Health Among Patients. J Prim Care Community Health 2022;13. https://doi.org/10.1177/21501319221113543. 21501319221113543.
95. Compton MT, Shim RS. The social determinants of mental health. Focus 2015; 13(4):419–25.
96. Muennig P, Schweinhart L, Montie J, et al. Effects of a prekindergarten educational intervention on adult health: 37-year follow-up results of a randomized controlled trial. Am J Public Health 2009;99(8):1431–7.
97. Schweinhart LJ, Montie JE, Xiang Z, et al. Lifetime Effects: The High/Scope Perry Preschool Study Through Age 40. High/Scope® Educational Research Foundation, 2005. Available at: https://nieer.org/wp-content/uploads/2014/09/specialsummary_rev2011_02_2.pdf (Accessed February 08, 23).

98. Campbell F, Conti G, Heckman JJ, et al. Early childhood investments substantially boost adult health. Science 2014;343(6178):1478–85.
99. Campbell FA, Pungello EP, Burchinal M, et al. Adult outcomes as a function of an early childhood educational program: an Abecedarian Project follow-up. Dev Psychol 2012;48(4):1033–43.
100. Muennig P, Robertson D, Johnson G, et al. The effect of an early education program on adult health: the Carolina Abecedarian Project randomized controlled trial. Am J Public Health 2011;101(3):512–6.
101. Karoly LA, Kilburn MR, Cannon JS. Early childhood interventions: proven results, Future Promise. Santa Monica, CA: RAND Corporation; 2005. Available at: https://www.rand.org/pubs/monographs/MG341.html. Accessed January 26, 2023.
102. Tanner AE, Palakshappa D, Morse CG, et al. Exploring the consequences of food insecurity and harnessing the power of peer navigation and mHealth to reduce food insecurity and cardiometabolic comorbidities among persons with HIV: protocol for development and implementation trial of weCare/Secure. Trials 2022;23(1):998.
103. Myers CA. Food Insecurity and Psychological Distress: a Review of the Recent Literature. Curr Nutr Rep 2020;9(2):107–18.
104. Gonyea JG, O'Donnell AE, Curley A, et al. Food insecurity and loneliness amongst older urban subsidised housing residents: The importance of social connectedness. Health Soc Care Community 2022;30(6):e5959–67.
105. Oronce CIA, Miake-Lye IM, Begashaw MM, et al. Interventions to Address Food Insecurity Among Adults in Canada and the US: A Systematic Review and Meta-analysis. JAMA Health Forum 2021;2(8):e212001.
106. Santilli A, Lin-Schweitzer A, Morales SI, et al. Coalition Building and Food Insecurity: How an Equity and Justice Framework Guided a Viable Food Assistance Network. Int J Environ Res Public Health 2022;19(18):11666.
107. Cummins S, Flint E, Matthews SA. New neighborhood grocery store increased awareness of food access but did not alter dietary habits or obesity. Health Aff 2014;33(2):283–91.
108. Thornton RL, Glover CM, Cené CW, et al. Evaluating Strategies For Reducing Health Disparities By Addressing The Social Determinants Of Health. Health Aff 2016;35(8):1416–23.
109. Ezeh A, Oyebode O, Satterthwaite D, et al. The history, geography, and sociology of slums and the health problems of people who live in slums. Lancet 2017; 389(10068):547–58.
110. World Health Organization. WHO guidance to protect health from climate change through health adaptation planning. Available at: https://www4.unfccc.int/sites/NAPC/Documents/Supplements/WHO%20H-NAP%202014.pdf. (Accessed January 26, 2023).
111. TenBrink DS, McMunn R, Panken S. Project U-Turn: increasing active transportation in Jackson, Michigan. Am J Prev Med 2009;37(6 Suppl 2):S329–35.
112. Ludwig J, Sanbonmatsu L, Gennetian L, et al. Neighborhoods, obesity, and diabetes–a randomized social experiment. N Engl J Med 2011;365(16):1509–19.
113. Ludwig J, Duncan GJ, Gennetian LA, et al. Neighborhood effects on the long-term well-being of low-income adults. Science 2012;337(6101):1505–10.
114. Gauld R, Blank R, Burgers J, et al. The World Health Report 2008 - Primary Healthcare: How Wide Is the Gap between Its Agenda and Implementation in 12 High-Income Health Systems? Healthc Policy 2012;7(3):38–58.

115. Dupre ME, George LK, Liu G, et al. The cumulative effect of unemployment on risks for acute myocardial infarction. Arch Intern Med 2012;172(22):1731–7.
116. Kaplan GA, Ranjit N, Burgard SA. Lifting gates, lengthening lives: did civil rights policies improve the health of African American woman in the 1960s and 1970s?. In: Schoeni RF, House JS, Kaplan GA, et al, editors. Making Americans healthier: social and economic policy as health policy. New York (NY): Russell Sage Foundation; 2008. p. 145–69.
117. Arno PS, House JS, Viola D, et al. Social security and mortality: the role of income support policies and population health in the United States. J Public Health Policy 2011;32(2):234–50.
118. Costello EJ, Erkanli A, Copeland W, et al. Association of family income supplements in adolescence with development of psychiatric and substance use disorders in adulthood among an American Indian population. JAMA 2010;303(19):1954–60.
119. Pega F, Pabayo R, Benny C, et al. Unconditional cash transfers for reducing poverty and vulnerabilities: effect on use of health services and health outcomes in low- and middle-income countries. Cochrane Database Syst Rev 2022;3(3):CD011135.
120. Dunne T, Bishop L, Avery S, et al. A Review of Effective Youth Engagement Strategies for Mental Health and Substance Use Interventions. J Adolesc Health 2017;60(5):487–512.
121. Smith ML, Steinman LE, Casey EA. Combatting Social Isolation Among Older Adults in a Time of Physical Distancing: The COVID-19 Social Connectivity Paradox. Front Public Health 2020;8:403.
122. Kawachi I, Colditz GA, Ascherio A, et al. A prospective study of social networks in relation to total mortality and cardiovascular disease in men in the USA. J Epidemiol Community Health 1996;50(3):245–51.
123. Doobay-Persaud A, Adler MD, Bartell TR, et al. Teaching the Social Determinants of Health in Undergraduate Medical Education: a Scoping Review. J Gen Intern Med 2019;34(5):720–30.
124. Thomas PA, Kern DE, Hughes MT, et al. Curriculum development for medical education: a six-step approach. Baltimore, MD: Johns Hopkins University Press; 2015.
125. Reeve K, Rossiter K, Risdon C. The Last Straw! A board game on the social determinants of health. Med Educ 2008;42(11):1125–6.
126. Harper AC. A proposal to incorporate a public health perspective into clinical teaching. Clin Teach 2011;8(2):114–7.
127. Erlich M, Blake R, Dumenco L, et al. Health disparity curriculum at the Warren Alpert Medical School of Brown University. R I Med J 2014;97(9):22–5.
128. Doran KM, Kirley K, Barnosky AR, et al. Developing a novel Poverty in Healthcare curriculum for medical students at the University of Michigan Medical School. Acad Med 2008;83(1):5–13.
129. Brown P.C., Roediger P.C. III, McDaniel M.A., Make It Stick, The science of successful learning, 2014, Belknap Press; Cambridge, MA.
130. Aronson L. Twelve tips for teaching reflection at all levels of medical education. Med Teach 2011;33(3):200–5.
131. Mezirow J. Fostering critical reflection in adulthood: a guide to transformative and emancipatory learning. San Francisco, CA: Jossey-Bass Publishers; 1991.
132. Cranton P. Understanding and promoting transformative learning: a guide to theory and practice. 3rd edition. Virginia, VA: Stylus Publishing; 2016.

133. Gottlieb LM, Wing H, Adler NE. A Systematic Review of Interventions on Patients' Social and Economic Needs. Am J Prev Med 2017;53(5):719–29.
134. Fichtenberg C, Delva J, Minyard K, et al. Health And Human Services Integration: Generating Sustained Health And Equity Improvements. Health Aff 2020; 39(4):567–73.
135. Fichtenberg CM, Alley DE, Mistry KB. Improving Social Needs Intervention Research: Key Questions for Advancing the Field. Am J Prev Med 2019;57(6 Suppl 1):S47–54.
136. Steketee G, Ross AM, Wachman MK. Health Outcomes and Costs of Social Work Services: A Systematic Review. Am J Public Health 2017;107(S3): S256–66.

Monitoring Social Determinants of Health Assessing Patients and Communities

Vincent Morelli, MD[a,*], Robert Joseph Heizelman, MD[b]

KEYWORDS

- Social determinants of health • Stress surveys • Geomapping • Biomarkers
- Z codes

KEY POINTS

- Surveys of social determinants of health (SDoH) are recommended by the Academy of Family Physicians, American Academy of Pediatrics, and other primary care organizations.
- A full exploration of SDoH is needed because they interconnected.
- Written or web-based survey formats are preferred by patients.
- A team based approach to screening is preferred, with the primary care provider reviewing screening findings.
- Blood and genetic tests for markers of chronic stress exist, but due to the current state of the research are not yet ready for clinical use.

MONITORING SOCIAL DETERMINANTS OF HEALTH

Social determinants of health (SDoH) are conditions in the environments where people are born, live, learn, work, play, worship, and age that affect a wide range of health, functioning, and quality-of-life outcomes and risks.[1] These determinants can have a powerful impact on individual health and well-being. In light of this, the Centers for Medicare and Medicaid Services (CMS) now recommends evaluating and monitoring SDoH in primary care encounters—this includes collecting SDoH data, documenting it in patient health records, assigning Z codes to encounters (see below), justifying

[a] Department of Family and Community Medicine, Meharry Medical College, 3rd Floor, Old Hospital Building, 1005 Dr. D. B. Todd, Jr., Boulevard, Nashville, TN 37208-3599, USA; [b] Department of Family Medicine, Medical Informatics, University of Michigan, 3rd Floor, Old Hospital Building, 1005 Dr. D. B. Todd, Jr., Boulevard, Nashville, TN 37208-3599, USA
* Corresponding author.
E-mail address: Morellivincent@gmail.com

Prim Care Clin Office Pract 50 (2023) 527–547
https://doi.org/10.1016/j.pop.2023.04.005

patient care and referral via use of these codes, and reporting Z codes to CMS in order to inform public health and policy research.[2]

From a clinical point of view, if we are to assist those whose lives are affected by suboptimal SDoH then we must be able to measure and quantify the stress arising from these determinants. Although we are not yet able to reliably do so, research is moving us in the right direction. There are at least 3 common methods of screening and monitoring used by researchers today—surveys; geomapping and biomarkers; and reporting via Z codes. We will discuss all below, first looking at surveys designed to assess individual stress exposure, then examining the role of geomapping and finally evaluating 3 of the commonly used biomarkers in the evaluation of stress and SDoH: interleukin 6 (IL6), cortisol, and epigenetic methylation. A final section on Z codes will look at the reporting of SDoH. It is intended that these approaches will become more accurate and clinically useful as research in the field progresses.

STRESS/SOCIAL DETERMINANTS OF HEALTH SURVEYS

Stress surveys, including those modeled after the 1967 Holmes and Raphe *Schedule of Recent Experiences Social Readjustment Rating Scale,*[3] have been in use for some time. These and other self-reported surveys[4–6] were developed by researchers in attempts to correlate health outcomes with stressful life events. However, to date, none of these surveys have been validated—as they rely on the subjective interpretation of stressful events and are thus unable to capture the individual variations and complexities involved. Keep in mind that there are no gold standard/*objective* indicators of SDoH against that we can reliably compare *subjective* SDoH survey results. Internal validation on the other hand, measured by Cronbach's alpha, indicates that similar survey items align (ie, if people who report being heavier also report bigger pant size or if they report conflicting answers).

In addition to these inconsistency barriers, primary care providers (PCPs) may also have ethical hesitations to survey screening. For example, screening and creating expectations of available assistance may seem unethical to PCPs who are not prepared to guarantee effective evidence-based interventions and referrals.[7,8] Cultural barriers, too, must be considered and providers may not feel adequately trained to approach all patients in our multicultural society. For example, it is important for PCPs be aware that some questions regarding race, income, or education may be perceived as prejudicial by racially disenfranchised populations. Or male providers with a superficial understanding of cultural issues may feel unsure in approaching female Muslim patients.

Despite these concerns, the American Academy of Pediatrics (AAP), the American Academy of Family Physicians, and the American College of Physicians all currently recommend SDoH surveillance[9,10] and monitoring—but without instructing how to screen or which assessment tool to use. On the AAP website alone, there are over 50 tool kits, website links, helplines, webinars, videos, fact sheets, reports, and articles addressing aspects of SDoH and vying for inclusion in clinical screening tools. It is not surprising then, that in practice such screening is rarely done. Even attuned pediatric clinics screen less than 25% of the time,[11] and fewer still close the loop by following referrals and outcomes.[12–14] The reason for the implementation gap, noted in roughly two-thirds of surveyed physicians, is a lack of time, resources, training, or compensation (see note below) [13,15] leaving most PCPs still unable or unwilling to adequately screen for stressful SDoH.[11] In light of this physician inability and reluctance, team-based screening, done by ancillary health workers (medical sssistants [MAs], registered nurses [RNs], etc.), has been recommended.[14,16] However, this approach still does not surmount the any of the survey shortcomings discussed above.

NOTE: The new January 2021 E/M billing codes now allow for 2 methods of billing. The first is a new time-based method of coding that will always allow for increased compensation based on increased physician time spent with patients or while coordinating care (level 3 = 30–44 minutes; level 4 = 45–59 minutes; level 5 = 60–74 minutes; add 99,417 for each 15 minutes beyond this). The second is a new medical-decision-making model necessitating the documentation of 2 of the following 3 elements: (1) number and complexity of problems addressed; (2) amount or complexity of data reviewed and analyzed; and (3) risk of complications/morbidity or mortality. Such billing changes allow for more comprehensive examination of SDoH and allow for increasing coding and billing. [9]

To date, there is no validated "best" set of SDoH screening surveys available for use in clinical practice, nor are there guidelines on how clinicians might best use the information collected for patient care and/or referral.[17,18] Although not abandoning the search for improved surveys, these inherent shortcomings have led researchers to look for other ways of quantifying stress and SDoH, bringing us to our other 2 methods of assessment: geomapping and biomarkers.

GEOMAPPING

A Geographic Information System (GIS) is a database of information that can be used to create, analyze, map, and visually display geographically referenced information. With respect to SDoH, there are several GIS that can identify both community characteristics and community resources. Examples include the Population Health Assessment Engine (PHATE) (https://dashboard.primeregistry.org/), FindHelp (https://go.findhelp.com), and the Southern Community Cohort Study (https://www.southerncommunitystudy.org/).

PHATE is a GIS tool commissioned by the American Board of Family Medicine and developed in collaboration with the Center for Applied Research and Engagement Systems at the University of Missouri. It utilizes publicly available census tract data to characterize communities based on a social deprivation index (SDI), as measured by 7 area-level deprivation characteristics including: percentage living in poverty, percentage with less than 12 years of education, percentage of single-parent households, percentage living in rented housing units, percentage living in overcrowded housing units, percentage of households without a car, and percentage of unemployed adults under age 65 years. Scoring the SDI results in a community vital sign (CVS)—a number between 0 and 100 that quantifies deprivation with respect to SDoH, with a higher score suggesting greater community deprivation.[19]

NOTE: Four pieces of information are required to determine the CVS via PHATE. These include street address, city, state, and zip code. Once this information has been entered, the GIS software returns census tract level data in a CVS color-coded score, red indicating a CVS of 81 to 100, orange 61 to 80, yellow 41 to 60, light green 21 to 40, and dark green indicating a CVS of 1 to 20. The breakdown of SDI domains is listed adjacently in table format that gives a better understanding of the community characteristics involved (**Fig. 1**).

Most studies using GIS mapping in relation to health do so using static census tract data, correlating health outcomes with zip codes. Findings can then be used to propose building new green spaces, providing more accessible health care, or making healthy foods or transportation more accessible. This is all valuable on the aggregate level but might be less useful on an individual patient level.[20–22]

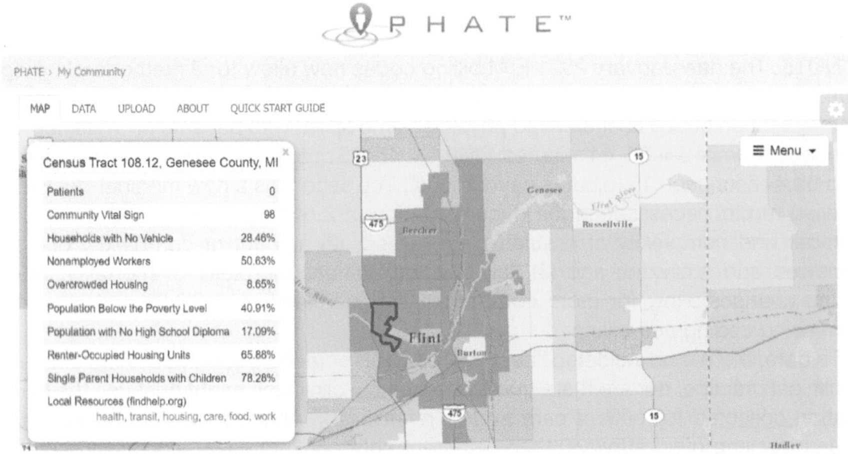
PHATE™
PHATE › My Community
MAP DATA UPLOAD ABOUT QUICK START GUIDE
Census Tract 108.12, Genesee County, MI
Patients 0
Community Vital Sign 98
Households with No Vehicle 28.46%
Nonemployed Workers 50.63%
Overcrowded Housing 8.65%
Population Below the Poverty Level 40.91%
Population with No High School Diploma 17.09%
Renter-Occupied Housing Units 65.88%
Single Parent Households with Children 78.28%
Local Resources (findhelp.org)
health, transit, housing, care, food, work
≡ Menu
Flint
Genesee
Russellville
Burton
Beecher

Fig. 1. PHATE. (*Courtesy of* Center for Applied Research and Engagement Systems (CARES), University of Missouri.)

For example, PCPs wishing to monitor the effect of "rurality" (associated with drug and alcohol use, depression from social isolation, etc.) on patients might better be served by surveying a patient's "activity space," noting not only where a patient resides, but also where they work, travel, and spend leisure time.[23] The activity space profile might then be used to focus patient encounter questions on related health issues like depression, drug and alcohol use, or exposure to workplace toxins.

BIOMARKERS

Background: the Concept of Inflammation as it Relates to Age, Disease, and Social Determinants of Health

Both aging and environmental stress have been documented to lower immune responsiveness, raise levels of circulating inflammatory mediators, and set the stage for the development of the chronic diseases of aging.[17,24] As such, inflammation is now accepted as the most significant driver of morbidity and mortality today, implicated as the underlying mechanism in over 50% of global deaths.[25,26] Because of this, recent research has focused on finding inflammatory biomarkers that might be easily and reliably measured and monitored with a goal of preventing morbidity from cardiovascular disease, cancer, metabolic syndrome, diabetes, fatty liver disease, autoimmune diseases, psychologic afflictions, neurodegenerative disorders, and all of the other stress related diseases of aging.[22–29]

In contrast to the acute stress reaction that is beneficially adaptative, chronic stress is detrimental, leading to the activation of immune mediators (eg, chemokines, cytokines), oxidative insult and deleterious changes at the cellular level, including DNA damage, telomere defects, epigenetic changes (see below), glycosylation of proteins, etc.[30,31] These cellular changes eventually manifest as "system-wide immune overload" contributing to the age-related maladies stated above.

Such chronic stress and the induced inflammatory and cellular changes have been documented to be brought on by social determinants including, stressful work environments, low level of education, exposure to environmental toxins, suboptimal built environments (contributing to obesity, smoking, alcohol and drug use, sleep disturbances, poor dietary habits, etc.), low socioeconomic status (SES), and an insufficient social network (resulting in loneliness, neglect, abuse, stressful romantic relationships, perceived discrimination, etc.).[32–43]

Exposure to these stressors often begins early in development (even in utero) and can persist through childhood creating inflammatory alterations that can eventually manifest as adult physical, mental, or behavioral afflictions.[44–46] However, one does not have to wait until adulthood to see the negative effects of stress. Infants born into households with low SES, documented to have higher levels of inflammatory markers at birth, have been found to display emotional and behavioral deficits when assessed at age 2 years.[47] Similar associations can be seen in the psychologic and cognitive profiles of adolescents—with stress adversely affecting things like executive function, episodic memory, and verbal fluency—all issues that can be further exacerbated in a vicious cycle by concomitant depression, obesity, substance use, or physical inactivity[48] which themselves can be brought on by other suboptimal SDoH.

The end result of detrimental SDoH is chronic stress, chronic inflammation, the disease manifestations mentioned above, and, importantly, a decreased ability to confront new stressors as they arise.[49–51] With this brief background regarding the role of stress and inflammation in disease, let us look at a few of the biomarkers commonly used in research today. This is by no means a comprehensive review, but rather is a sampling, meant to give the PCP an idea of the complexities involved with assessing biomarkers and a lens through which to view future advancements in the field.

Individual Biomarker Indicators of Inflammation

There are well over 25 commonly monitored proteins that are indicative of ongoing inflammation. They can be divided into at least 7 major categories: cytokines, adhesion molecules, growth factors, chemokines, metalloproteinases, liver-produced inflammatory agents, and neutrophil activation.[52] Below we will examine one primary mediator of stress (the cytokine, interleukin 6 [IL 6]), one commonly used hormonal stress marker (cortisol), and one indicator of inflammation at the cellular level (epigenetic methylation of DNA or histone proteins). Following this, we will look at the work being done in regard to constructing "composite stress scores" that might better monitor suboptimal SDoH and might prove more accurate predictors of their resultant physical and psychologic disease states.

Interleukin 6: A Primary Mediator of Stress

IL-6 is a circulating nonspecific marker of inflammation that, in response to insult by stress, infection, or environmental exposure, is released from CD4 lymphocytes, monocytes, damaged endothelial cells, and adipocytes. It can induce a harmful cytokine cascade, signaling autoimmune and inflammatory responses that have been associated with chronic infection, diabetes, atherosclerosis, depression, systemic lupus erythematosus, multiple myeloma, prostate cancer, rheumatoid arthritis, stroke, and other conditions.[53–61] Because of the fact that IL-6 induces the release of C-reactive protein (CRP) from the hepatocytes, IL-6 and CRP are often studied together when speaking of inflammatory markers—IL-6 usually seen as primary.

The widespread effect of IL-6 is due to its effect on several target tissues including hepatocytes (causing the synthesis and release of CRP, serum amyloid A, fibrinogen, hepcidin, and inhibiting albumin synthesis) and bone (increasing both osteoblastic and osteoclastic activity and increasing platelet production). IL-6 can cause epigenetic changes as well (see later discussion), including methylating DNA, altering gene expression, and leading to premature cellular aging.[62–64]

In terms of SDoH, those with low SES have been found to have higher levels of circulating IL-6 (and CRP)[58,59] – a factor felt to play a role in the higher incidence of morbidity and mortality from myocardial infarction, stroke, heart failure and other related conditions. IL6 disease associations in this setting have been documented to be independent of other covariates such as behavioral risk factors, psychosocial stressors or environmental toxins.[37,44,65–70]

Despite this known association, there are several issues involved with using IL-6 as a marker for SDoH in clinical practice. First, IL-6 measurements can be influenced by several factors including exercise,[71] diet,[54,72,73] supplementation,[74] and other coexisting medical conditions. For example, in the case of exercise, IL-6 blood levels may increase up to a 100-fold. However, in this case, IL-6 is *not* an indicator of inflammation rather, due to complex factors, it acts in a beneficial way *protecting against* systemic inflammation. Dietary factors too can affect IL-6 measurements with omega 3s, curcumin, probiotics, whole grains, and others known to lower IL-6, whereas sugar and high fat intake known to do the reverse.

The second issue involved in IL-6 measurement is the fact that IL-6 is an unstable plasma protein subject to strict collection and handling requirements. It must be centrifuged within 30 minutes with the separated plasma then measured (or frozen) within 24 hours. Thirdly, and perhaps most importantly, is that there is no universally accepted reference range for what constitutes a normal serum IL-6 level—what is normal in one individual may be abnormal in another.

The above is likely more than we need to know in the clinical setting, but it gives us insight into the difficulties that arise with monitoring many of the cytokines, chemokines, and neutrophil activators relevant in inflammation. Suffice it to say that due to difficulties posed by complex and confounding factors as well as strict collection and handling requirements, IL-6 and other cytokines remain less than ideal markers for inflammation in the clinical setting.

Cortisol: A Hormonal Stress Marker

The hypothalamic–pituitary–adrenal (HPA) axis normally reacts to stress by releasing cortisol, promoting gluconeogenesis, and generally contributing to the fight-or-flight signals that ready the body for adaptation and action. Usually this beneficial HPA response returns to baseline once the stressful event has passed. In the case of chronic unrelenting stress however, the "event" remains unresolved and, as a result, the homeostatic system is overloaded leading to the many harmful effects brought on by persistently high circulating cortisol. Such effects include degradation of muscle protein, enhanced osteoclastic activity, hippocampal memory and learning deficits, central adiposity, hypertension, and a "burned out" immune systems unable to fight off future infection or other inflammatory disease. Much like a patient with chronic obstructive pulmonary disease on long-term exogenous corticosteroids, patients with chronic stress and chronically high cortisol exhibit a suppressed HPA axis, making them less able to mount an adequate stress response in the face of new insults.[75–77]

Research hoped that cortisol levels would be a reasonable choice as a biomarker—an indicator of stress and inflammation that could be easily measured and used clinically. However, as with IL-6, cortisol is not quite yet ready for prime time. To understand why, we must first look briefly at the normal physiology of the hormone.

Normally, cortisol release peaks in the morning 30 to 45 minutes after awakening, followed by a gradual diurnal decline to a nadir at around midnight.[78] However, within this normal diurnal variation, both intra-individual and inter-individual differences exist, making interpretation of levels difficult.[79,80] Further complicating interpretation is the fact that many other factors such as sleep, exercise, mental state,[81–83] environment,[84] medications,[85,86] and diet[87] to name a few, have all been proven to affect levels. In addition, depending on the level and duration of the stress involved, the HPA can display either hyper- or hypoactivation.[88] with different types of stressors (physical neglect vs. emotional abuse) affecting the HPA axis and cortisol levels differently.[89]

One promising insight (although not yet useful in the clinical setting) is that when researchers measured cortisol levels over time, they noted the *shape* of the declining cortisol curve to be significant—generally finding that cortisol curves with a sharp decline (higher peaks and quicker drop-offs) were associated with better physical and psychosocial health[79] whereas those with blunted response curves (lower peaks and slower drop offs) were less salutary.[90] Despite promise, however, studies to date have documented conflicting results in this regard and must undergo further examination before clinical usefulness can be established.[91,92]

Another recent promising approach was thought to be the measurement of hair cortisol concentration (HCC). Much like hemoglobin A1c measures average glucose levels over a 3 month period, HCC was thought to provide a retrospective look at cortisol levels over time. As hair grows at an average of 1 cm/mo, it was felt that a snapshot of a patient's cortisol level, for example, 6 months ago, was possible by sampling hair 6 cm from the scalp.[93] Here again measurement and interpretation were fraught with difficulties. First was the fact that hair growth rates vary with age, gender, ethnicity and hair thickness,[94,95] making standardization of normal levels difficult. In addition, male and older subjects and those with a higher body mass index (BMI) were all found to have higher HCC, necessitating adjustment for age, sex and weight. Mental states (eg, anxiety, depression, bipolar disease, post-traumatic stress disorder) were also found to influence levels and to vary not only with the illness itself, but also with age of onset and duration of illness.[93] HCC was also found to vary with athletic status, shift work, underemployment, and chronic pain.[96] And finally, hair was found to have lower cortisol concentrations toward the distal ends of hairs, suggesting that some chemical dissolution was taking place over time. Thus, on top of all of the other confounding variables mentioned above, adjustments in interpretation of results would have to be made for this falling concentration in longer hairs.[85]

In sum, as with the cytokine IL-6, the hormone cortisol is burdened with a multitude of difficulties in measurement and a similar stable of confounding variables. Comparable difficulties are found with the other less studied biomarkers. These shortcomings have led researchers to look for more stable measures of chronic stress and inflammation. One new area that holds promise is epigenetics.

Epigenetics: A Cellular Level Stress INDICATOR

Epigenetics, the nurture side of inheritance, provides a link between the environment including stress,[97] socioeconomic status, work,[98] diet,[99] smoking, air pollution, particulate matter,[100] and the genome. When environmental factors reach critical levels, inflammation can induce chemical alterations—either on DNA itself or on the histone proteins that surround and support DNA in the cell nucleus. These alterations can affect gene expression (turning genes on or off), alter protein transcription (increase or decrease important enzymes such as those involved in lipolysis or gluconeogenesis), and result in adaptive or maladaptive cellular and organism level changes. Not only can such epigenetic changes affect the organism involved, but they are also heritable, meaning that organisms can pass on these DNA or histone alterations to their offspring—in essence passing on epigenetic adaptation to the environment.[101–104]

One of the most extensively studied epigenetic alterations is methylation—either of DNA itself or of the supporting histone proteins.[105] (NOTE: The reader may come across "chromatin methylation" in the literature, the definition of chromatin being, "a complex of nucleic acids and proteins, primarily histones, in the cell nucleus. Histones can be modified in many ways besides methylation, including acetylation, phosphorylation, adenylation, and ubiquitination, all of which affect the transcriptional activity of genes.[106] These changes have been noted but have been less studied.)

Such methylation, brought on by stress, is followed by altered genetic expression and protein transcription, resulting in (often) harmful downstream target tissue alterations. Much as with inflammation, these alterations have demonstrated roles in numerous conditions including gastrointestinal, thyroid and other cancers,[107–110] psychiatric conditions,[111] rheumatologic diseases,[112] hypertension, cardiovascular disease,[113,114] and other age-related diseases such as osteoarthritis and osteoporosis.[115] Methylation has also been shown to affect memory and learning,[116,117] and to represent a remarkably accurate "aging clock," establishing a biological age capable of predicting mortality much more accurately than chronologic age (or of other risk scoring systems such as the Framingham risk score).[118]

On top of the role that epigenetics play in DNA replication, repair, aging, and disease, of particular interest to researchers is the fact that epigenetic changes are reversible, making them potential sites for intervention and manipulation—either by environmental alteration or drug targeting.[119,120] Such intervention is being made easier by advancing knowledge. For example, of the 20+ million possible methylation sites on the human genome, just a few thousand sites have been documented where DNA methylation is closely correlated with disease and age-related issues.[121] Monitoring these specific areas, rather than the entire genome, allows researchers to focus their efforts when measuring an organism's response to stress or when contemplating intervention. Focusing on patterns of methylation at these sites holds promise in early cancer detection, therapeutic intervention and monitoring.[120,122]

Again, Difficulties in Measuring

In clinical practice, most *DNA sampling* today is done from whole blood, red blood cells, cell-free DNA (fragments of DNA circulating in the blood outside of the cell), or saliva.[123] *Histone methylation*, on the other hand, is measured more globally as total methyl content.[124] As with the other biomarkers discussed above, collecting, measuring, and standardizing normal ranges in regard to epigenetic markers is complicated.

First, one must account for epigenetic changes are dynamic and subject to the vagaries of a changing environment, including both exacerbating and protective factors. Proven protective factors mitigating the chronic stress associated with suboptimal SDoH include exercise,[125,126] relaxation techniques,[127] dietary habits such as restricted calorie intake or carbohydrates restriction, probiotics,[128–130] as well as the "epigenetic diet"—a corollary of the Mediterranean Diet that includes the consumption of foods such as whole grains, soy, cruciferous, and other vegetables, omega-3 fatty acids, fruit, legumes, extra virgin olive oil, fresh fish, and a moderate consumption of red wine—proven to protect against cancer and other diseases, and to be associated with longevity and reduced all-cause mortality.[131–134]

Second, the methylation data sought may be "tissue specific." Sampling is usually done from a proxy tissue such as whole blood, the assumption being that the methylation in blood cells is similar to that of the tissue in question. This can obviously be problematic as methylation patterns in the blood may not accurately reflect that of the target tissue.[123,135]

Additionally, there are many different types of blood cells in whole blood, each with the possibility of slightly different methylation content, adding to the measurement variability (single-cell epigenetics circumvents this issue). There are also difficulties establishing rigorous "normal" levels of methylation, with the testing of tissue samples, and with statistical methods of quantifying alterations—each aspect requiring consideration of covariates such as smoking, BMI, etc. that will affect methylation. Finally, although the reliability of measurements across labs has been demonstrated, minor alterations in subtype methylation and differences with different types of lab equipment have been acknowledged.[124,136–139]

In addition to the practical considerations above, ethical questions and privacy challenges must be addressed. What should the PCP do with disease predicting data if inadvertently found when monitoring for SDoH? Who has rights to the data? How much responsibility do we have for those living with suboptimal SDoH? And how active must we be in advocating for change? All of these, and other questions, will have to be considered as we move forward.

Although the study of DNA and histone methylation is in its nascent stages, its potential to impact the monitoring and prevention of disease is highlighted in the last 5 years alone over 30,000 articles have been published in the field. As with the other biomarkers discussed above, epigenetic researchers agree that they have only begun to illuminate the intricacies of epigenetics and unlock their clinical utility.[118]

Composite Biomarker Scores as Indicators of Inflammation and Disease

Because of the limitations in measuring and monitoring individual biomarkers, in recent years, researchers have begun exploring if combinations of biomarkers that might be more useful “composite score” indicators of chronic stress and SDoH. In the next section, we will look at 2 commonly discussed composite scores. This is not meant to be an exhaustive review, but rather a sampling to give PCPs a literacy in the field and an idea of what the future may hold.

The Concept of Allostatic Load

One of the common composite scoring systems used in the discussion of chronic stress and SDoH is the idea of allostatic load. The term was introduced in the literature by McEwen and Stellar in 1993[140] and was defined as “the wear and tear” on the body caused by chronic stress. [141,142] Since then, researchers have been trying to reliably measure the cumulative effect of chronic stress via an allostatic load composite score. In contrast to “single inflammatory marker scientists,” allostatic load researchers attempt to construct a score formulated from 2 categories of chronic stress indicators: primary *mediators* of stress (eg, cortisol, epinephrine, IL-6, other inflammatory cytokines) arising from alterations in the autonomic nervous system or HPA system; and secondary *indicators* of stress (eg, CVD, blood pressure, waist circumference, HBA1c) manifesting in measurable health parameters.[143,144]

In theory, this seemed reasonable—an organism attempting to maintain homeostasis in the face of chronic stress, inducing measurable changes in their primary and secondary markers, contributing to their allostatic load composite score and finally to health and disease outcomes. Again however, in practice, such scoring has yet to prove reliable, clinically useful, or statistically validated. As with inflammation research, allostatic load researchers have yet to come to a consensus on (1) *what* to measure (besides the more commonly used 25 markers mentioned above, several others have been used or proposed); (2) *when and how* to measure them (as with primary inflammatory biomarkers, secondary indicators too are subject to diurnal variations, temporal changes with aging, alterations with patient medication, supplement use, physical condition, mental state, diet, environmental conditions, etc.); (3) what normal reference ranges are; (4) how individual markers of allostatic load might best be combined into a useful, validated, allostatic load composite score; (5) which individual markers should be weighted more in scoring. This is important in the face of a genetic propensity for specific diseases. Should cortisol be weighted more when looking at those with a family history of diabetes? Should inflammatory cytokines be weighted more in those with a genetic bent toward cardiovascular disease?; and (6) how allostatic load markers should be modified in the face of protective factors like strong social networks, exercise, or a "future focused" attitude.[145–154]

Despite these limitations, and despite the fact that we have yet to find a clinically useful allostatic load scoring system, when we look at it from a broader perspective, the concept is an important one to keep in mind as research across 3 decades has demonstrated allostatic load's impact on health outcomes including cardiovascular disease, functional decline, frailty, sarcopenia, dental disease, and substance use.[81,155–160]

Cumulative Biologic Risk

Another composite score that the reader may come across in the literature is the cumulative biologic risk (CBR) score. CBR has been utilized as a comprehensive measure of risk across at least 4 physiologic systems (usually cardiovascular, metabolic, inflammatory, and neuroendocrine) using an array of biomarkers. For example, studies have measured CBR of (1) the cardiovascular system via systolic blood pressure, diastolic blood pressure, and resting heart rate; (2) the metabolic system via hemoglobin A1c, fasting total cholesterol-HDL cholesterol ratio, and waist circumference; (3) the inflammatory system via white blood cell count; and (4) the neuroendocrine system via serum cortisol. (Other studies[161] have used additional indicators such as body mass index, glomerular filtration rate, serum albumen. Still others[162] have added obesity as a measure of SES, educational attainment and income levels.)

Underpinning CBR is the reasonable notion that the 4 physiologic systems work in concert when influencing disease pathogenesis, synergistically amplifying or attenuating risk. However, as with allostatic load, CBR is fraught with individual biomarker measurement and interpretation difficulties and with difficulties in constructing composite score measurements. Again, we are given a useful lens through which to view disease pathogenesis but to date, no standardized, universally accepted composite CBR has proven useful in the clinical setting.[163–165]

Z CODES: REPORTING SOCIAL DETERMINANTS OF HEALTH

Z codes are ICD-10 uncompensated secondary billing codes intended to capture SDoH that are used in addition to primary patient diagnosis codes. Although the use of Z codes has increased since their inception in 2015, they are still only documented in 1.4% of Medicare/Medicaid visits.[166] This is largely due to 2 factors. First, the coding is not compensated by CMS or other insurers, and second because the codes were initially tailored more toward social workers rather than PCPs. These issues persist despite attempts by CMS to clarify that the codes could be used by any clinician involved in patient care.[167] From a researcher's perspective, this undercoding is disheartening, leaving them unable to estimate the full impact of SDoH on disease burden, health care utilization, and general health-system repercussions.[168]

In the future, if we are to increase Z code use and reporting, codes will have to be standardized across providers and financial incentives will likely have to be instituted.[169] As research in the field advances it is hoped that a weighted prioritization of SDoH or perhaps the creation of critical "SDoH clusters" will be uncovered, resulting in composite Z codes that will be more useful for reporting, patient care, referral (eg, findhelp.organd portal.networkofcare.org), PCP compensation,[169] and the monitoring of SDoH.

CASE STUDY

As one may have surmised from reading the above, we are not yet clinically ready to monitor SDoH via inflammatory markers, cortisol, epigenetic changes, aging clocks, or composite biomarker scores. However, just this kind of monitoring will likely be possible in the near future, as researchers are making significant inroads in this direction.[170] Until this time, PCPs might think in reverse. For example, using a pediatric patient presenting with asthma as a "canary in a coal mine," indicating a need for GIS screening to assess for risk factors associated with the recent rise in asthma rates in impoverished neighborhoods. Such screening might reveal high areas of poverty, public housing, or violent crime—all prompting referral to appropriate agencies with the knowledge that if these SDoH are not addressed, they will lead to further long-term health, education, and income disparities.[171] Similarly, poor academic performance in adolescent patients should prompt a need to probe deeper for social determinants of learning—covert physical, mental or psychosocial health issues, and detrimental built, social or economic environments.[172]

DISCUSSION

Despite the challenges of measuring and monitoring SDoH, research in the field is at an admirable early stage. Researchers must start somewhere and measure something if they are to help clinicians, public health workers, and policymakers assess and intervene. In the future, it is likely that combinations of stress-survey data,[4,173,174] geomapping, biomarker measurements, and other factors will be incorporated into an advanced inflammatory/SDoH composite score.[175]

This will likely occur with an assist from machine learning,[176,177] hopefully allowing PCPs to predict, intervene, and monitor patient health and to help direct public-health workers and policymakers to improve individual and societal health.[25,178]

If we are to make advances against the greatest health challenge of our time, we must incorporate consideration of SDoH into our primary care visits—suspecting involvement, being ready to assess the immediate and long-term medical needs arising therefrom, having a patient-friendly referral networks ready, and using systems to monitor compliance and effect.

CLINICS CARE POINTS

- When screening, the PCP should be aware of the cultural issues that may be involved.
- Written or web-based survey formats are preferred by patients.
- Addressing one determinant may have little effect without addressing others—a full exploration of all SDoH is needed because of their interconnectedness.
- PCPs should be ready to refer with a full and accessible referral network.

REFERENCES

1. Healthy People 2030, U.S. Department of Health and Human Services, Office of Disease Prevention and Health Promotion. Available at: https://health.gov/healthypeople/objectives-and-data/social-determinants-health Accessed January 22, 2023.
2. Centers for Medicare and Medicaid Services. USING Z CODES: The Social Determinants of Health (SDOH). Available at: https://www.cms.gov/files/document/zcodes-infographic.pdf). Accessed July 01, 2023.
3. Holmes TH, Rahe RH. The Social Readjustment Rating Scale. J Psychosom Res 1967;11(2):213–8.

4. Dohrenwend BS, Krasnoff L, Askenasy AR, et al. Exemplification of a method for scaling life events: the Peri Life Events Scale. J Health Soc Behav 1978;19(2):205–29.
5. Gray MJ, Litz BT, Hsu JL, et al. Psychometric properties of the life events checklist. Assessment 2004;11(4):330–41.
6. Chang Weir, Rosy et al. Incorporating Social Drivers of Health Data into Risk Stratification Models to Address Health Inequities: Defining the PRAPARE Stakeholder-Vetted Risk Stratification Model, June 3, 2022 . Available at: https://prapare.org/knowledge-center/whitepapers-and-publications/prapare-risk-stratification-principles/. Accessed January 18, 23.
7. Garg A, Boynton-Jarrett R, Dworkin PH. Avoiding the Unintended Consequences of Screening for Social Determinants of Health. JAMA 2016;316(8):813–4.
8. Finkelhor D. Screening for adverse childhood experiences (ACEs): Cautions and suggestions. Child Abuse Negl 2018;85:174–9.
9. American Academy of Family Physicians. The EveryONE Project. Available at: https://www.aafp.org/patient-care/social-determinants-of-health/everyone-project.html. Accessed February, 2023.
10. American Academy of Pediatrics. Social Determinants of Health Screening Resources. https://www.aap.org/en/patient-care/screening-technical-assistance-and-resource-center/screening-resource-library/social-determinants-of-health/?page=1&sortDirection=1&sortField=Year. Accessed 02 01, 23.
11. Friedman S, Caddle S, Motelow JE, et al. Improving Screening for Social Determinants of Health in a Pediatric Resident Clinic: A Quality Improvement Initiative. Pediatr Qual Saf 2021;6(4):e419.
12. Patel M, Bathory E, Scholnick J, et al. Resident documentation of social determinants of health: effects of a teaching tool in the outpatient setting. Clin Pediatr (Phila) 2018;57:451–6.
13. Morgenlander MA, Tyrrell H, Garfunkel LC, et al. Screening for Social Determinants of Health in Pediatric Resident Continuity Clinic. Acad Pediatr 2019;19(8):868–74.
14. Chung EK, Siegel BS, Garg A, et al. Screening for Social Determinants of Health Among Children and Families Living in Poverty: A Guide for Clinicians. Curr Probl Pediatr Adolesc Health Care 2016;46(5):135–53.
15. Leavitt Partners. "Taking Action on Social Determinants of Health" Report, October 22, 2019. https://leavittpartners.com/press/leavitt-partners-releases-taking-action-on-social-determinants-of-health-report/. Accessed 01 08, 23.
16. O'Gurek DT, Henke C. A Practical Approach to Screening for Social Determinants of Health. Fam Pract Manag 2018;25(3):7–12.
17. Gottlieb LM, Francis DE, Beck AF. Uses and Misuses of Patient- and Neighborhood-level Social Determinants of Health Data. Perm J 2018;22:18–078.
18. National Academies of Sciences, Engineering, and Medicine. Integrating social care into the Delivery of health care: moving Upstream to improve the Nation's health. Washington, DC: The National Academies Press; 2019. https://doi.org/10.17226/25467.
19. Butler DC, Petterson S, Phillips RL, et al. Measures of social deprivation that predict health care access and need within a rational area of primary care service delivery. Health Serv Res 2013;48(2 Pt 1):539–59.

20. Warren JC, Smalley KB. In: Warren JC, editor. Rural public health: best practices and preventive models. New York: Springer Publishing Company; 2014. p. 11–28.
21. Alfero C, Barnhart T, Berrsch D, et al. P] Brief. National Rural Health Association; 2013. The future of rural health; p. 26. Available at: https://www.ruralhealth.us/getattachment/Advocate/Policy-Documents/FutureofRuralHealthFeb-2013.pdf.aspx?lang=en-US. Accessed March 18, 23.
22. Coomber K, Toumbourou JW, Miller P, et al. Rural adolescent alcohol, tobacco, and illicit drug use: a comparison of students in Victoria, Australia, and Washington State, United States. J Rural Health 2011;27(4):409–15.
23. Mao L, Stacciarini JM, Smith R, et al. An individual-based rurality measure and its health application: A case study of Latino immigrants in North Florida, USA. Soc Sci Med 2015;147:300–8.
24. Furman D, Chang J, Lartigue L, et al. Expression of specific inflammasome gene modules stratifies older individuals into two extreme clinical and immunological states. Nat Med 2017;23(2):174–84.
25. Furman D, Campisi J, Verdin E, et al. Chronic inflammation in the etiology of disease across the life span. Nat Med 2019;25(12):1822–32.
26. Burska AN, Sakthiswary R, Sattar N. Effects of Tumour Necrosis Factor Antagonists on Insulin Sensitivity/Resistance in Rheumatoid Arthritis: A Systematic Review and Meta-Analysis. PLoS One 2015;10(6):e0128889.
27. GBD 2017 Causes of Death Collaborators. Global, regional, and national age-sex-specific mortality for 282 causes of death in 195 countries and territories, 1980-2017: a systematic analysis for the Global Burden of Disease Study 2017. Lancet 2018;392(10159):1736–88. https://doi.org/10.1016/S0140-6736(18)32203-7 [published correction appears in Lancet. 2019;393(10190):e44] [published correction appears in Lancet. 2018 Nov 17;392(10160):2170].
28. Proctor MJ, McMillan DC, Horgan PG, et al. Systemic inflammation predicts all-cause mortality: a glasgow inflammation outcome study. PLoS One 2015;10(3):e0116206.
29. Xi Y, Lin Y, Guo W, et al. Multi-omic characterization of genome-wide abnormal DNA methylation reveals diagnostic and prognostic markers for esophageal squamous-cell carcinoma. Signal Transduct Target Ther 2022;7(1):53.
30. Campisi J. Aging, cellular senescence, and cancer. Annu Rev Physiol 2013;75:685–705.
31. Franceschi C, Garagnani P, Parini P, et al. Inflammaging: a new immune-metabolic viewpoint for age-related diseases. Nat Rev Endocrinol 2018;14(10):576–90.
32. Zitvogel L, Pietrocola F, Kroemer G. Nutrition, inflammation and cancer. Nat Immunol 2017;18(8):843–50.
33. Razzoli M, Nyuyki-Dufe K, Gurney A, et al. Social stress shortens lifespan in mice. Aging Cell 2018;17(4):e12778.
34. Yuan J, Liu Y, Wang J, et al. Long-term Persistent Organic Pollutants Exposure Induced Telomere Dysfunction and Senescence-Associated Secretary Phenotype. J Gerontol A Biol Sci Med Sci 2018;73(8):1027–35.
35. Kennedy BK, Berger SL, Brunet A, et al. Geroscience: linking aging to chronic disease. Cell 2014;159(4):709–13.
36. Chandola T, Brunner E, Marmot M. Chronic stress at work and the metabolic syndrome: prospective study. BMJ 2006;332(7540):521–5.

37. Iyer HS, Hart JE, James P, et al. Impact of neighborhood socioeconomic status, income segregation, and greenness on blood biomarkers of inflammation. Environ Int 2022;162:107164.
38. Burini RC, Anderson E, Durstine JL, et al. Inflammation, physical activity, and chronic disease: An evolutionary perspective. Sports Med Health Sci 2020; 2(1):1–6.
39. Loprinzi PD. Health Behavior Combinations and Their Association with Inflammation. Am J Health Promot 2016;30(5):331–4.
40. Mullington JM, Simpson NS, Meier-Ewert HK, et al. Sleep loss and inflammation. Best Pract Res Clin Endocrinol Metab 2010;24(5):775–84.
41. Shields GS, Slavich GM. Lifetime Stress Exposure and Health: A Review of Contemporary Assessment Methods and Biological Mechanisms. Soc Personal Psychol Compass 2017;11(8):e12335.
42. Donoho CJ, Crimmins EM, Seeman TE. Marital Quality, Gender, and Markers of Inflammation in the MIDUS Cohort. J Marriage Fam 2013;75(1):127–41.
43. Robles TF, Slatcher RB, Trombello JM, et al. Marital quality and health: a meta-analytic review. Psychol Bull 2014;140(1):140–87.
44. Miller GE, Chen E, Parker KJ. Psychological stress in childhood and susceptibility to the chronic diseases of aging: moving toward a model of behavioral and biological mechanisms. Psychol Bull 2011;137(6):959–97.
45. Natale BN, Manuck SB, Shaw DS, et al. Systemic Inflammation Contributes to the Association Between Childhood Socioeconomic Disadvantage and Midlife Cardiometabolic Risk. Ann Behav Med 2023;57(1):26–37.
46. Fleming TP, Watkins AJ, Velazquez MA, et al. Origins of lifetime health around the time of conception: causes and consequences. Lancet 2018;391(10132): 1842–52.
47. Pham C, Bekkering S, O'Hely M, et al. Infant inflammation predicts childhood emotional and behavioral problems and partially mediates socioeconomic disadvantage [published online ahead of print, 2022 May 23]. Brain Behav Immun 2022;104:83–94.
48. Mac Giollabhui N, Hartman CA. Examining inflammation, health, stress and lifestyle variables linking low socioeconomic status with poorer cognitive functioning during adolescence [published online ahead of print, 2022 Apr 28]. Brain Behav Immun 2022;104:1–5.
49. Kotas ME, Medzhitov R. Homeostasis, inflammation, and disease susceptibility. Cell 2015;160(5):816–27.
50. Shen-Orr SS, Furman D, Kidd BA, et al. Defective Signaling in the JAK-STAT Pathway Tracks with Chronic Inflammation and Cardiovascular Risk in Aging Humans. Cell Syst 2016;3(4):374–84.e4.
51. Bennett JM, Reeves G, Billman GE, et al. Inflammation-Nature's Way to Efficiently Respond to All Types of Challenges: Implications for Understanding and Managing "the Epidemic" of Chronic Diseases. Front Med 2018;5:316.
52. Kuban KC, O'Shea TM, Allred EN, et al. The breadth and type of systemic inflammation and the risk of adverse neurological outcomes in extremely low gestation newborns. Pediatr Neurol 2015;52(1):42–8.
53. Tackey E, Lipsky PE, Illei GG. Rationale for interleukin-6 blockade in systemic lupus erythematosus. Lupus 2004;13(5):339–43.
54. Milesi G, Rangan A, Grafenauer S. Whole Grain Consumption and Inflammatory Markers: A Systematic Literature Review of Randomized Control Trials. Nutrients 2022;14(2):374.

55. Gadó K, Domján G, Hegyesi H, et al. Role of INTERLEUKIN-6 in the pathogenesis of multiple myeloma. Cell Biol Int 2000;24(4):195–209.
56. Smith PC, Hobisch A, Lin DL, et al. Interleukin-6 and prostate cancer progression. Cytokine Growth Factor Rev 2001;12(1):33–40.
57. Nishimoto N. Interleukin-6 in rheumatoid arthritis. Curr Opin Rheumatol 2006; 18(3):277–81.
58. Zhu H, Wang Z, Yu J, et al. Role and mechanisms of cytokines in the secondary brain injury after intracerebral hemorrhage. Prog Neurobiol 2019;178:101610.
59. Kristiansen OP, Mandrup-Poulsen T. Interleukin-6 and diabetes: the good, the bad, or the indifferent? Diabetes 2005;54(Suppl 2):S114–24.
60. Dowlati Y, Herrmann N, Swardfager W, et al. A meta-analysis of cytokines in major depression. Biol Psychiatry 2010;67(5):446–57.
61. Xu Z, Wang W, Liu Q, et al. Association between gaseous air pollutants and biomarkers of systemic inflammation: A systematic review and meta-analysis. Environ Pollut 2022;292(Pt A):118336.
62. Foran E, Garrity-Park MM, Mureau C, et al. Upregulation of DNA methyltransferase-mediated gene silencing, anchorage-independent growth, and migration of colon cancer cells by interleukin-6. Mol Cancer Res 2010; 8(4):471–81.
63. Muscatell KA, Brosso SN, Humphreys KL. Socioeconomic status and inflammation: a meta-analysis. Mol Psychiatry 2020;25(9):2189–99.
64. Lam PH, Chiang JJ, Chen E, et al. Race, socioeconomic status, and low-grade inflammatory biomarkers across the lifecourse: A pooled analysis of seven studies. Psychoneuroendocrinology 2021;123:104917.
65. Addo J, Ayerbe L, Mohan KM, et al. Socioeconomic status and stroke: an updated review. Stroke 2012;43(4):1186–91.
66. Kaptoge S, Seshasai SR, Gao P, et al. Inflammatory cytokines and risk of coronary heart disease: new prospective study and updated meta-analysis. Eur Heart J 2014;35(9):578–89.
67. Hawkins NM, Jhund PS, McMurray JJ, et al. Heart failure and socioeconomic status: accumulating evidence of inequality. Eur J Heart Fail 2012;14(2):138–46.
68. Alter DA, Chong A, Austin PC, et al. Socioeconomic status and mortality after acute myocardial infarction. Ann Intern Med 2006;144(2):82–93.
69. Nusslock R, Miller GE. Early-Life Adversity and Physical and Emotional Health Across the Lifespan: A Neuroimmune Network Hypothesis. Biol Psychiatry 2016;80(1):23–32.
70. Danese A, McEwen BS. Adverse childhood experiences, allostasis, allostatic load, and age-related disease. Physiol Behav 2012;106(1):29–39.
71. Pedersen BK, Febbraio MA. Muscle as an endocrine organ: focus on muscle-derived interleukin-6. Physiol Rev 2008;88(4):1379–406.
72. Custodero C, Mankowski RT, Lee SA, et al. Evidence-based nutritional and pharmacological interventions targeting chronic low-grade inflammation in middle-age and older adults: A systematic review and meta-analysis. Ageing Res Rev 2018;46:42–59.
73. Derosa G, Maffioli P, Simental-Mendía LE, et al. Effect of curcumin on circulating interleukin-6 concentrations: A systematic review and meta-analysis of randomized controlled trials. Pharmacol Res 2016;111:394–404.
74. Zhai J, Bo Y, Lu Y, et al. Effects of Coenzyme Q10 on Markers of Inflammation: A Systematic Review and Meta-Analysis. PLoS One 2017;12(1):e0170172.
75. Chrousos GP. Stress and disorders of the stress system. Nat Rev Endocrinol 2009;5:374–81.

76. Sheridan MA, How J, Araujo M, et al. What are the links between maternal social status, hippocampal function, and HPA axis function in children? Dev Sci 2013; 16(5):665–75.
77. Hajat A, Diez-Roux A, Franklin TG, et al. Socioeconomic and race/ethnic differences in daily salivary cortisol profiles: the multi-ethnic study of atherosclerosis. Psychoneuroendocrinology 2010;35(6):932–43.
78. Pruessner JC, Wolf OT, Hellhammer DH, et al. Free cortisol levels after awakening: a reliable biological marker for the assessment of adrenocortical activity. Life Sci 1997;61(26):2539–49.
79. Adam EK, Hawkley LC, Kudielka BM, et al. Day-to-day dynamics of experience–cortisol associations in a population-based sample of older adults. Proc Natl Acad Sci U S A 2006;103(45):17058–63.
80. De Nys L, Anderson K, Ofosu EF, et al. The effects of physical activity on cortisol and sleep: A systematic review and meta-analysis. Psychoneuroendocrinology 2022;143:105843.
81. Juster RP, McEwen BS, Lupien SJ. Allostatic load biomarkers of chronic stress and impact on health and cognition. Neurosci Biobehav Rev 2010;35(1):2–16.
82. Zorn JV, Schür RR, Boks MP, et al. Cortisol stress reactivity across psychiatric disorders: A systematic review and meta-analysis. Psychoneuroendocrinology 2017;77:25–36.
83. Joseph NT, Jiang Y, Zilioli S. Momentary emotions and salivary cortisol: A systematic review and meta-analysis of ecological momentary assessment studies. Neurosci Biobehav Rev 2021;125:365–79.
84. Antonelli M, Barbieri G, Donelli D. Effects of forest bathing (shinrin-yoku) on levels of cortisol as a stress biomarker: a systematic review and meta-analysis. Int J Biometeorol 2019;63(8):1117–34.
85. Stalder T, Steudte-Schmiedgen S, Alexander N, et al. Stress-related and basic determinants of hair cortisol in humans: A meta-analysis. Psychoneuroendocrinology 2017;77:261–74.
86. Sahebkar A, Rathouska J, Simental-Mendía LE, et al. Statin therapy and plasma cortisol concentrations: A systematic review and meta-analysis of randomized placebo-controlled trials. Pharmacol Res 2016;103:17–25.
87. Gibson EL, Checkley S, Papadopoulos A, et al. Increased salivary cortisol reliably induced by a protein-rich midday meal. Psychosom Med 1999;61(2): 214–24.
88. Khoury JE, Bosquet Enlow M, Plamondon A, et al. The association between adversity and hair cortisol levels in humans: A meta-analysis. Psychoneuroendocrinology 2019;103:104–17.
89. Bruce J, Fisher PA, Pears KC, et al. Morning cortisol Levels in preschool-aged foster children: differential effects of maltreatment type. Dev Psychobiol 2009; 51(1):14–23.
90. Brindle RC, Pearson A, Ginty AT. Adverse childhood experiences (ACEs) relate to blunted cardiovascular and cortisol reactivity to acute laboratory stress: A systematic review and meta-analysis. Neurosci Biobehav Rev 2022;134:104530.
91. Bremner JD, Vythilingam M, Vermetten E, et al. Cortisol response to a cognitive stress challenge in posttraumatic stress disorder (PTSD) related to childhood abuse. Psychoneuroendocrinology 2003;28(6):733–50.
92. Wessa M, Rohleder N, Kirschbaum C, et al. Altered cortisol awakening response in posttraumatic stress disorder. Psychoneuroendocrinology 2006; 31(2):209–15.

93. Stalder T, Kirschbaum C. Analysis of cortisol in hair–state of the art and future directions. Brain Behav Immun 2012;26(7):1019–29.
94. Harkey MR. Anatomy and physiology of hair. Forensic Sci Int 1993;63(1–3):9–18.
95. Van Neste DJ, Rushton DH. Gender differences in scalp hair growth rates are maintained but reduced in pattern hair loss compared to controls. Skin Res Technol 2016;22(3):363–9.
96. Staufenbiel SM, Penninx BW, Spijker AT, et al. Hair cortisol, stress exposure, and mental health in humans: a systematic review. Psychoneuroendocrinology 2013; 38(8):1220–35.
97. Sosnowski DW, Booth C, York TP, et al. Maternal prenatal stress and infant DNA methylation: A systematic review. Dev Psychobiol 2018;60(2):127–39.
98. Freni-Sterrantino A, Fiorito G, D'Errico A, et al. Work-related stress and well-being in association with epigenetic age acceleration: A Northern Finland Birth Cohort 1966 Study. Aging (Albany NY) 2022;14(3):1128–56.
99. Kadayifci FZ, Zheng S, Pan YX. Molecular Mechanisms Underlying the Link between Diet and DNA Methylation. Int J Mol Sci 2018;19(12):4055.
100. Ferrari L, Carugno M, Bollati V. Particulate matter exposure shapes DNA methylation through the lifespan. Clin Epigenetics 2019;11(1):129.
101. Mattei AL, Bailly N, Meissner A. DNA methylation: a historical perspective. Trends Genet 2022;38(7):676–707.
102. Horváth V, Merenciano M, González J. Revisiting the Relationship between Transposable Elements and the Eukaryotic Stress Response. Trends Genet 2017;33(11):832–41.
103. Law PP, Holland ML. DNA methylation at the crossroads of gene and environment interactions. Essays Biochem 2019;63(6):717–26.
104. Tan Q. Epigenetic age acceleration as an effective predictor of diseases and mortality in the elderly. EBioMedicine 2021;63:103174.
105. Li E, Zhang Y. DNA methylation in mammals. Cold Spring Harb Perspect Biol 2014;6(5):a019133.
106. Audia JE, Campbell RM. Histone Modifications and Cancer. Cold Spring Harb Perspect Biol 2016;8(4):a019521.
107. Zhou W, Dinh HQ, Ramjan Z, et al. DNA methylation loss in late-replicating domains is linked to mitotic cell division. Nat Genet 2018;50(4):591–602.
108. Zafon C, Gil J, Pérez-González B, et al. DNA methylation in thyroid cancer. Endocr Relat Cancer 2019;26(7):R415–39.
109. Berman BP, Weisenberger DJ, Aman JF, et al. Regions of focal DNA hypermethylation and long-range hypomethylation in colorectal cancer coincide with nuclear lamina-associated domains. Nat Genet 2011;44(1):40–6.
110. Greger V, Passarge E, Höpping W, et al. Epigenetic changes may contribute to the formation and spontaneous regression of retinoblastoma. Hum Genet 1989; 83(2):155–8.
111. Klengel T, Pape J, Binder EB, et al. The role of DNA methylation in stress-related psychiatric disorders. Neuropharmacology 2014;80:115–32.
112. Ciechomska M, Roszkowski L, Maslinski W. DNA Methylation as a Future Therapeutic and Diagnostic Target in Rheumatoid Arthritis. Cells 2019;8(9):953.
113. Xia Y, Brewer A, Bell JT. DNA methylation signatures of incident coronary heart disease: findings from epigenome-wide association studies. Clin Epigenetics 2021;13(1):186.
114. Joáo Job PM, Dos Reis Lívero FA, Junior AG. Epigenetic Control of Hypertension by DNA Methylation: A Real Possibility. Curr Pharm Des 2021;27(35): 3722–8.

115. Salameh Y, Bejaoui Y, El Hajj N. DNA Methylation Biomarkers in Aging and Age-Related Diseases. Front Genet 2020;11:171.
116. Heyward FD, Sweatt JD. DNA Methylation in Memory Formation: Emerging Insights. Neuroscientist 2015;21(5):475–89.
117. Klemp I, Hoffmann A, Müller L, et al. DNA methylation patterns reflect individual's lifestyle independent of obesity. Clin Transl Med 2022;12(6):e851. https://doi.org/10.1002/ctm2.851.
118. Alpert A, Pickman Y, Leipold M, et al. A clinically meaningful metric of immune age derived from high-dimensional longitudinal monitoring. Nat Med 2019;25(3):487–95.
119. Chang WL, Hsieh CH, Kuo IY, et al. Nutlin-3 acts as a DNA methyltransferase inhibitor to sensitize esophageal cancer to chemoradiation. Mol Carcinog 2023;62(2):277–87.
120. Ren L, Yang Y, Li W, et al. Recent advances in epigenetic anticancer therapeutics and future perspectives. Front Genet 2023;13:1085391. https://doi.org/10.3389/fgene.2022.1085391.
121. Horvath S, Raj K. DNA methylation-based biomarkers and the epigenetic clock theory of ageing. Nat Rev Genet 2018;19(6):371–84.
122. Talukdar FR, Soares Lima SC, Khoueiry R, et al. Genome-Wide DNA Methylation Profiling of Esophageal Squamous Cell Carcinoma from Global High-Incidence Regions Identifies Crucial Genes and Potential Cancer Markers. Cancer Res 2021;81(10):2612–24.
123. Husby A. On the Use of Blood Samples for Measuring DNA Methylation in Ecological Epigenetic Studies. Integr Comp Biol 2020;60(6):1558–66.
124. Singer BD. A Practical Guide to the Measurement and Analysis of DNA Methylation. Am J Respir Cell Mol Biol 2019;61(4):417–28.
125. Ren H, Collins V, Clarke SJ, et al. Epigenetic changes in response to tai chi practice: a pilot investigation of DNA methylation marks. Evid Based Complement Alternat Med 2012;2012:841810.
126. White AJ, Sandler DP, Bolick SC, et al. Recreational and household physical activity at different time points and DNA global methylation. Eur J Cancer 2013;49(9):2199–206.
127. Pavanello S, Campisi M, Tona F, et al. Exploring Epigenetic Age in Response to Intensive Relaxing Training: A Pilot Study to Slow Down Biological Age. Int J Environ Res Public Health 2019;16(17):3074.
128. Carlberg C, Velleuer E. Nutrition and epigenetic programming. Curr Opin Clin Nutr Metab Care 2022. https://doi.org/10.1097/MCO.0000000000000900 [published online ahead of print, 2022 Dec 26].
129. Cordero P, Campion J, Milagro FI, et al. Leptin and TNF-alpha promoter methylation levels measured by MSP could predict the response to a low-calorie diet. J Physiol Biochem 2011;67(3):463–70.
130. Shock T, Badang L, Ferguson B, et al. The interplay between diet, gut microbes, and host epigenetics in health and disease. J Nutr Biochem 2021;95:108631. https://doi.org/10.1016/j.jnutbio.2021.108631.
131. Kenanoglu S, Gokce N, Akalin H, et al. Implication of the Mediterranean diet on the human epigenome. J Prev Med Hyg 2022;63(2 Suppl 3):E44–55.
132. Sapienza C, Issa JP. Diet, Nutrition, and Cancer Epigenetics. Annu Rev Nutr 2016;36:665–81.
133. Andreescu N, Puiu M, Niculescu M. Effects of Dietary Nutrients on Epigenetic Changes in Cancer. Methods Mol Biol 2018;1856:121–39.

134. Divella R, Daniele A, Savino E, et al. Anticancer Effects of Nutraceuticals in the Mediterranean Diet: An Epigenetic Diet Model. Cancer Genomics Proteomics 2020;17(4):335–50.
135. Gunasekara CJ, Scott CA, Laritsky E, et al. A genomic atlas of systemic interindividual epigenetic variation in humans. Genome Biol 2019;20(1):105.
136. Fischer MA, Vondriska TM. Clinical epigenomics for cardiovascular disease: Diagnostics and therapies. J Mol Cell Cardiol 2021;154:97–105.
137. Nestor C, Ruzov A, Meehan R, et al. Enzymatic approaches and bisulfite sequencing cannot distinguish between 5-methylcytosine and 5-hydroxymethylcytosine in DNA. Biotechniques 2010;48(4):317–9.
138. Wilhelm-Benartzi CS, Koestler DC, Karagas MR, et al. Review of processing and analysis methods for DNA methylation array data. Br J Cancer 2013;109(6): 1394–402.
139. Zhang Y, Baheti S, Sun Z. Statistical method evaluation for differentially methylated CpGs in base resolution next-generation DNA sequencing data. Brief Bioinform 2018;19(3):374–86.
140. McEwen BS, Stellar E. Stress and the individual. Mechanisms leading to disease. Arch Intern Med 1993;153(18):2093–101.
141. Franceschi C, Campisi J. Chronic inflammation (inflammaging) and its potential contribution to age-associated diseases. J Gerontol A Biol Sci Med Sci 2014; 69(Suppl 1):S4–9.
142. Stepanova M, Rodriguez E, Birerdinc A, et al. Age-independent rise of inflammatory scores may contribute to accelerated aging in multi-morbidity. Oncotarget 2015;6(3):1414–21.
143. Seeman TE, McEwen BS, Rowe JW, et al. Allostatic load as a marker of cumulative biological risk: MacArthur studies of successful aging. Proc Natl Acad Sci U S A 2001;98(8):4770–5.
144. Juster RP, Bizik G, Picard M, et al. A transdisciplinary perspective of chronic stress in relation to psychopathology throughout life span development. Dev Psychopathol 2011;23(3):725–76.
145. Gruenewald TL, Seeman TE, Ryff CD, et al. Combinations of biomarkers predictive of later life mortality. Proc Natl Acad Sci U S A 2006;103(38):14158–63.
146. Karlamangla AS, Singer BH, McEwen BS, et al. Allostatic load as a predictor of functional decline. MacArthur studies of successful aging. J Clin Epidemiol 2002;55(7):696–710.
147. Seplaki CL, Goldman N, Glei D, et al. A comparative analysis of measurement approaches for physiological dysregulation in an older population. Exp Gerontol 2005;40(5):438–49.
148. Seplaki CL, Goldman N, Weinstein M, et al. Measurement of cumulative physiological dysregulation in an older population. Demography 2006;43(1):165–83.
149. Dowd JB, Simanek AM, Aiello AE. Socio-economic status, cortisol and allostatic load: a review of the literature. Int J Epidemiol 2009;38(5):1297–309.
150. Juster RP, Marin MF, Sindi S, et al. Allostatic load associations to acute, 3-year and 6-year prospective depressive symptoms in healthy older adults. Physiol Behav 2011;104(2):360–4.
151. Piazza JR, Almeida DM, Dmitrieva NO, et al. Frontiers in the use of biomarkers of health in research on stress and aging. J Gerontol B Psychol Sci Soc Sci 2010; 65(5):513–25.
152. Loucks EB, Juster RP, Pruessner JC. Neuroendocrine biomarkers, allostatic load, and the challenge of measurement: A commentary on Gersten. Soc Sci Med 2008;66(3):525–30.

153. Chen E, Miller GE, Lachman ME, et al. Protective factors for adults from low-childhood socioeconomic circumstances: the benefits of shift-and-persist for allostatic load. Psychosom Med 2012;74(2):178–86 [published correction appears in Psychosom Med. 2015 Apr;77(3):344] [published correction appears in Psychosom Med. 2015 Apr;77(3):344].
154. Gholami A, Baradaran HR, Hariri M. Can soy isoflavones plus soy protein change serum levels of interlukin-6? A systematic review and meta-analysis of randomized controlled trials. Phytother Res 2021;35(3):1147–62.
155. Beckie TM. A systematic review of allostatic load, health, and health disparities. Biol Res Nurs 2012;14(4):311–46.
156. Leahy R, Crews DE. Physiological dysregulation and somatic decline among elders: modeling, applying and re-interpreting allostatic load. Coll Antropol 2012;36(1):11–22.
157. Poulton R, Caspi A, Milne BJ, et al. Association between children's experience of socioeconomic disadvantage and adult health: a life-course study. Lancet 2002;360(9346):1640–5.
158. Picca A, Coelho-Junior HJ, Calvani R, et al. Biomarkers shared by frailty and sarcopenia in older adults: A systematic review and meta-analysis. Ageing Res Rev 2022;73:101530.
159. Guidi J, Lucente M, Sonino N, et al. Allostatic Load and Its Impact on Health: A Systematic Review. Psychother Psychosom 2021;90(1):11–27.
160. Gallo LC, Fortmann AL, Mattei J. Allostatic load and the assessment of cumulative biological risk in biobehavioral medicine: challenges and opportunities. Psychosom Med 2014;76(7):478–80.
161. Talegawkar SA, Jin Y, Kandula NR, et al. Associations between Cumulative Biological Risk and Subclinical Atherosclerosis in Middle- and Older-Aged South Asian Immigrants in the United States. J Asian Health 2021;1(1):e202104.
162. Doom JR, Mason SM, Suglia SF, et al. Pathways between childhood/adolescent adversity, adolescent socioeconomic status, and long-term cardiovascular disease risk in young adulthood. Soc Sci Med 2017;188:166–75.
163. King KE, Morenoff JD, House JS. Neighborhood context and social disparities in cumulative biological risk factors. Psychosom Med 2011;73(7):572–9.
164. Merkin SS, Basurto-Dávila R, Karlamangla A, et al. Neighborhoods and cumulative biological risk profiles by race/ethnicity in a national sample of U.S. adults: NHANES III. Ann Epidemiol 2009;19(3):194–201.
165. Barber S, Hickson DA, Kawachi I, et al. Neighborhood Disadvantage and Cumulative Biological Risk Among a Socioeconomically Diverse Sample of African American Adults: An Examination in the Jackson Heart Study. J Racial Ethn Health Disparities 2016;3(3):444–56.
166. Heidari E, Zalmai R, Richards K, et al. Z-code documentation to identify social determinants of health among Medicaid beneficiaries. Res Social Adm Pharm 2023;19(1):180–3.
167. Center for Medicare and Medicaid Services. ICD-10-CM Official guidelines for coding and reporting, FY 2018. Baltimore, MD, 2018. Available at: https://www.cms.gov/medicare/coding/icd10/downloads/2018-icd-10-cm-coding-guidelines.pdf. Accessed at 02 08, 23.
168. Agency for Healthcare Research. SDOH Resources. Available at: https://www.ahrq.gov/sdoh/resources.html. Accessed 02 11, 23.
169. Truong HP, Luke AA, Hammond G, et al. Utilization of Social Determinants of Health ICD-10 Z-Codes Among Hospitalized Patients in the United States, 2016-2017. Med Care 2020;58(12):1037–43.

170. Berg MT, Rogers EM, Riley K, et al. Incarceration exposure and epigenetic aging in neighborhood context. Soc Sci Med 2022;310:115273.
171. Harris KM. Mapping inequality: Childhood asthma and environmental injustice, a case study of St. Louis, Missouri. Soc Sci Med 2019;230:91–110.
172. Sanderson CD, Hollinger-Smith LM, Cox K. Developing a Social Determinants of Learning™ Framework: A Case Study. Nurs Educ Perspect 2021;42(4):205–11.
173. Repetti RL, Taylor SE, Seeman TE. Risky families: family social environments and the mental and physical health of offspring. Psychol Bull 2002;128(2):330–66.
174. Levenstein S, Prantera C, Varvo V, et al. Development of the Perceived Stress Questionnaire: a new tool for psychosomatic research. J Psychosom Res 1993;37(1):19–32.
175. Slopen N, Goodman E, Koenen KC, et al. Socioeconomic and other social stressors and biomarkers of cardiometabolic risk in youth: a systematic review of less studied risk factors. PLoS One 2013;8(5):e64418.
176. Rauschert S, Raubenheimer K, Melton PE, et al. Machine learning and clinical epigenetics: a review of challenges for diagnosis and classification. Clin Epigenetics 2020;12(1):51.
177. Tian Q, Zou J, Tang J, et al. MRCNN: a deep learning model for regression of genome-wide DNA methylation. BMC Genom 2019;20(Suppl 2):192.
178. Schüssler-Fiorenza Rose SM, Contrepois K, Moneghetti KJ, et al. A longitudinal big data approach for precision health. Nat Med 2019;25(5):792–804.

Health Equity and Access to Health Care as a Social Determinant of Health: The Role of the Primary Care Provider

Coleman Pratt, MD[a,*], Riley Taylor, MD, MPH[b], Stacy D. Smith, MD[c]

KEYWORDS

• Social determinants of health • Health • Health equity • Health inequity
• Primary care • Access to care • Structural inequality • Community health center

KEY POINTS

- Health equity is defined by all populations having an opportunity to achieve their highest level of health care.
- Social determinants of health and access to health care are key elements in achieving health equity.
- Both structural and clinical barriers to care affect health equity.
- The primary care physician plays a unique role in improving health equity.

CASE STUDY

Part 1: Assessment

A 51-year-old Hispanic woman who immigrated to the United States from Honduras 6 years ago and works as a house cleaner presents to clinic in a community health center complaining of low back pain. She has been reluctant to seek medical care because of cost and a language barrier. The clinic offers Saturday morning hours and is located on a bus route to provide enhanced access to care for working poor people.

The patient completes a PHQ-9 and scores a 14, indicating moderate depression. Her vitals are normal, other than a calculated BMI of 28.5. The Spanish speaking nurse screens the patient for Diabetes, discovering a non-fasting blood sugar of 114 and a Hemoglobin A1C of 6.0.

[a] Department of Family and Community Medicine, Tulane University School of Medicine, 1430 Tulane Avenue, #8033 New Orleans, LA 70112-2699, USA; [b] Department of Preventive Medicine, Cook County Health, 1950 West Polk Street, Chicago, IL 60612, USA; [c] Department of Family & Community Medicine, Meharry Medical College, 1005 Dr. D. B. Todd, Jr., Boulevard, Nashville, TN 37208-3599, USA
* Corresponding author.
E-mail address: cpratt2@tulane.edu

Prim Care Clin Office Pract 50 (2023) 549–559
https://doi.org/10.1016/j.pop.2023.04.006

Her intake evaluation reveals the patient is past due for breast, cervical, and colorectal screening. The nurse enters this information into the electronic health record which has prevention screening alerts enabled.

The physician has access to a medical assistant who is a certified medical translator who joins the visit, and she completes a history and physical examination with special attention paid to low back pain, the patient's depression, and the prediabetes revealed at intake.

Defining Health Equity

In a social context, equity can be defined as "the effort to provide different levels of support based on an individual's or group's needs to achieve fairness in outcomes."[1] Multiple entities have definitions for health equity. The Centers for Disease Control and Prevention (CDC) defines it as "the state in which everyone has a fair and just opportunity to attain their highest level of health." Healthy People 2030 definition is "the attainment of the highest level of health for all people."[2]

The World Health Organization defines health equity as being achieved when everyone can attain their full potential for health and well-being. Key to health equity is a focus on addressing societal factors to address injustices caused by social, economic, demographic, or geographic factors.[3]

The need for health equity is driven by health disparities. Health disparities, as defined by the CDC, are "preventable differences in the burden of disease, injury, violence, or opportunities to achieve optimal health that are experienced by populations that have been disadvantaged by their social or economic status, geographic location, and environment."[2]

Current State of Health Equity: Race and Ethnicity

Current data demonstrate that there is much work to be done to achieve health equity in the United States. Racial disparities exist in nearly every state. Overall, Black, American Indian, and Alaskan Native (AIAN) populations have worse health outcomes.[4]

Although Latin/Hispanic populations in general are less likely to die from preventable causes compared with black populations, trends in data show increasing mortality and increasing prevalence of chronic conditions among this population. Black and AIAN are also at higher risk for complications of diabetes, including death, than other populations. Black, Latinx/Hispanic, and AIAN adults are more likely to be uninsured than white adults, who are less likely to face cost-related barriers to health care.[5]

Although policy efforts like the Affordable Care Act have helped to increase access to insurance, gaps in coverage and negative health outcomes still disproportionately affect vulnerable populations.[4]

Current State of Health Equity: Structural Inequality

Root causes of health disparities are driven by structural inequities. Structural inequities are divisions in society that place certain groups of people within a population at a disadvantage. Examples of structural inequities include racism, sexism, classism, ableism, xenophobia, and homophobia.[6]

Historically in the United States racism has been a major driver in societal inequities and health disparities due to lasting effects of slavery, segregation, and continued structural factors. Black Americans have a lower life expectancy than White Americans and have higher rates of diseases such as diabetes, hypertension, obesity, asthma, and heart disease.[7]

Environmental factors have also historically been a source of structural inequality. Where people live is a social determinant of health that can lead to environmental exposures that lead to health disparities. Exposure to environmental pollutants in air and water can lead to health problems such as respiratory illnesses and even cancer. Factories or facilities that produce pollution are more likely to be positioned near poor neighborhoods due to the lack of voice or influence in political decisions.[8]

Employment is a social determinant of health not only due to its link to income and poverty but also because of its link to health insurance. Because the US health care system relies on employer-based health insurance, people who are unemployed or work jobs that do not provide them with health insurance are at a disadvantage.[9]

Current State of Health Equity: Vulnerable Populations

Structural inequities can leave certain vulnerable populations at higher risk for health problems due to worse access to care or worse quality of care compared with other populations. Broadly defined, a vulnerable population is any group of people "whose demographic, geographic, or economic characteristics impede or prevent their access to health care services".[10]

Impoverished populations

Health care inequity is often driven by poverty. Low income can lead to difficulty affording health insurance and other health care associated costs including medications. People living in poverty may not be able to afford healthy food or may only be able to afford to live in neighborhoods that are in food deserts lacking access to healthy foods or grocery stores. All of these factors lead to higher rates of mental illness, chronic disease, and mortality in impoverished communities.[11–13] For children, poverty is associated with developmental delays, toxic stress, chronic illness, and nutritional problems. The effects of childhood poverty on health can endure into adulthood and is associated with obesity, smoking, substance use, and chronic stress.[14]

Minority populations

Because of the impact of racism on social determinants of health, communities of color have experienced health inequities. Lasting impacts of slavery, segregation, and systemic racism have dictated where black individuals can live, work, play, and go to school, which then lead to environmental, social, and economic impacts on health. Data show that racial and ethnic minority groups have higher rates of diabetes, hypertension, obesity, asthma, heart disease, and death compared with white populations.[7]

Gender as a vulnerable population

Health outcomes can also be affected by gender inequalities. Gender norms can dictate the amount of access and control that women have over health-related resources such as reproductive health care. Women are also subject to gender bias from clinicians, leading to delays in diagnosing and treating cardiovascular disease and incomplete treatment of pain.[14]

Sexual and gender minorities also experience health inequities related to social determinants. Negative attitudes about lesbian gay bisexual transgender questioning (LGBTQ) populations can lead to discrimination, bullying, and violence that can have negative impacts on mental health. LGBTQ youth are at increased risk for mental health conditions including depression, suicide and substance use, and for sexual risk behaviors.[15] Trans individuals may face financial or social barriers to accessing desired gender-affirming medical treatment.[16]

Rural populations

Rural Americans are another vulnerable population subject to health disparities. People who live in rural areas are more likely to die from heart disease, cancer, and stroke.

Far distances to emergency health care services or specialists can impact access to care for this population. In addition, some rural areas may have exposure to specific environmental hazards that put them at higher risk for disease. Rural communities generally have higher rates of cigarette smoking, less physical activity, and lower use of seatbelts than in urban communities. All of these factors impact the inequitable health outcomes in these communities.[17]

Disabled populations

People with physical and intellectual disabilities face unique challenges in accessing health care. Physical accessibility to clinics and transportation can have a greater impact on access to care for these individuals. An increased risk of depression and anxiety is seen in this population. They also are more likely to smoke, and less likely to engage in physical activity, which are associated with poor health outcomes.[18]

Elderly populations

An increasing portion of the population, the elderly is also vulnerable to health inequities. Older adults are at higher risk for chronic health problems such as diabetes or heart disease, falls, and hospitalization for infection. Mobility issues in older adults can also limit their access to care.[19]

Mental health and substance using populations

People with mental health conditions and substance can also face challenges in accessing health care. Stigma and discrimination are social factors that impact ability and willingness to access care. In addition, people with mental health conditions may face barriers to employment and education. This puts people with mental health conditions at higher risk of disability and early death.[20]

CASE STUDY

Part 2: Intervention

The patient opts for a conservative approach to her back pain and agrees to trial a course of non steroidal anti inflamatories (NSAIDs) and to follow the Spanish language low back pain and weight loss educational information her physician provided. The patient declined medication for her prediabetes and depression. She agreed to meet with the behavioral health provider in clinic and follow her doctor's recommendation for increased cardiovascular exercise.

Before discharge, the physician reviews her prevention alerts and orders a mammogram and fecal immunochemical test (FIT) testing for the patient and schedules her to return in 2 weeks for follow-up and a pap smear.

At checkout, her lack of insurance is noted by the clerk and the patient is scheduled to see the Medicaid enrollment specialist when she returns for her follow-up visit in 2 weeks.

The patient returns in 2 weeks and reports that her back pain is improved and that her mood is slightly improved. She reports that she is finding the cognitive behavioral therapy (CBT) sessions with her therapist to be surprisingly beneficial.

The patient misses her follow-up visit at 3 months. Fortunately, the electronic health record (EHR) alerts the registered nurse case manager (RNCM) that the patient is past due to prevention screening and she calls the patient. The patient tells her that she did not know where to go for her mammogram and that she lost the instructions for her FIT testing.

The nurse sends the patient new FIT instructions in Spanish and helps her schedule her screening mammogram. The patient is instructed to consult the scheduling portal and pick a time that agrees with her work schedule for the follow-up visit.

ACCESS TO CARE

Access to health care is defined as "the timely use of health services to achieve the best health outcomes."[21] Equitable access to primary care and prevention services is one of the hallmarks of a successful health care system yielding better quality of care and lower overall cost. Studies from developed and underdeveloped countries have demonstrated that greater access to health care leads to better patient outcomes, decreased hospitalizations, and fewer emergency department visits.[22] Similar studies found that countries with greater emphasis on primary care had more success in mitigating the effects of income inequality and reducing socioeconomic disparities in access to health care.[23]

Barriers to health services exist on multiple levels encompassing systemic, provider, and patient-related factors. These barriers often result in delayed care or unmet health care needs. In a recent survey, patient's cited systemic-level barriers as most significant in impeding access to care almost twice as often as other types of accessibility barriers.[24] Systemic-level issues include cost of care, availability of insurance/adequate insurance coverage, transportation, number of clinics, and availability of providers. In contrast, provider-level barriers are those directly influenced by the provider–patient relationship. Decreased level of trust or confidence that patients have in their providers, language barriers, office wait times, and limited access to providers with adequate cultural competence of the populations they are serving are all examples of provider-level barriers to health care. The lack of access to care at the provider level has been linked to incidences of discrimination and bias resulting in delayed, impaired, or complete prevention of care.[25] Finally, problems accessing care at the individual level include issues such as inability to take time off from work, issues finding alternative childcare, or reliable transportation.[24]

In 2008 survey, systemic barriers and discrimination were found to have the greatest influence on perceived access to care. However, any combination of these barriers leads to unmet medical needs, delay of care, increased emergency room visits for preventable or nonemergent complaints, and increased financial burden on the individual and health care system as a whole.[24]

Roughly 30 million US residents are currently without health insurance. This includes 6.4 million that are eligible for Medicaid or Children's Health Insurance Program but not enrolled, 4.8 million living below the poverty level in Medicaid non-expansion states and 3.1 million undocumented immigrants.[26] The rate of uninsured is nearly double in states without Medicaid expansion, especially among minority groups.[27]

Even among those with health insurance, many report insufficient coverage resulting in delayed or inadequate care.[25] This holds particularly true for the elderly, many of whom suffer from limited mobility in addition to increasing cost of coverage gaps on fixed incomes which results in decreased access to outpatient clinics. In addition, women's health remains at the forefront of debate, especially concerning women's reproductive rights. With the repeal of Roe v Wade, access to abortion and family planning services has been significantly restricted in most Midwestern and Southern states. At present, 26 US states currently have or are in the process of enacting legislation aimed at criminalizing the act of performing abortions by imposing fines and felony charges to physicians providing the service.[28] These acts not only restrict access to abortion services from a geographic standpoint but also may negatively impacts the doctor–patient relationship.

Policy Change to Improve Access to Care

Over the past 20 years, there have been multiple health care policies and advancements in technology aimed at improving access to care among US residents. These efforts include but are not limited to (1) increased federal funding of community health care centers and safety net programs; (2) increased home visits for the elderly and chronically disabled; (3) increased utilization of telemedicine; and (4) the Affordable Care Act and Medicaid expansion programs.

Under the Affordable Care Act, over 17 million uninsured Americans were able to retain health care coverage over the last decade. Since its inception, the number of uninsured, non-elderly individuals decreased from 48.2 million in 2010 to 30.0 million individuals by the end of 2020.[29] The aim of this program is to provide improved quality of care and to lower the cost of health care by increasing public insurance options and through the expansion of Medicaid. As of March, 2023, 40 states have adopted and implemented Medicaid. North Carolina has adopted Medicaid expansion but has not yet implemented it, whereas 10 states, Wyoming, Kansas, Texas, Wisconsin, Tennessee, Mississippi, Alabama, Georgia, South Carolina, and Florida, have not adopted Medicaid Expansion.[30]

The enrollment eligibility was broadened to include individuals and families living at or below 138% of the federal poverty line (FPL). In those states that adopted expansion, the rate of uninsured individuals between the years of 2013 and 2016 dropped from 18.4% to 9.2%. The rate of uninsured has also declined in non-expansion states as well, which is partly attributable to the Affordable Care Act (ACA) market exchange premium subsidy.[27] Although the rate of uninsured in non-expansion state decreased from 22.7% to 17.9% between 2013 and 2016, the rate of uninsured in non-expansion states is nearly twice as high as those in expansion states.[29] The ACA has had significant impact on reducing racial and socioeconomic disparities in access to health care, but the percentage of non-Hispanic white US residents is still significantly lower than the rates of any other individual ethnic or minority group.[31] In addition, as of 2021, 12 states continued to oppose Medicaid expansion. Of those 12 states, 11 had the highest rate of uninsured residents in the nation.[27]

Clinical Strategies to Improve Access to Care

Since the early 2000s, community health care centers (CHCs) have emerged as an important resource for improving access to care for rural areas, lower income populations, and minority groups. Studies have found that increased presence of CHCs in communities is associated with lower rates of hospitalizations and emergency department visits for management of preventable nonemergent illness. Funding for these centers increased under the Health Center Program provision of the ACA and most recently through the Bipartisan Budget Act of 2018.[32] These centers provide primary care, behavioral health, and dental care to underserved communities.

For the elderly and those with chronic disabilities, home-based visits have proven to be invaluable. Individuals with limited mobility often have greater medical need but have fewer outpatient physician visits. JAMA Internal Medicine conducted a study showing that over 2 million Medicare recipients aged 65 years or older were homebound in 2011.[33] This patient population was found to have significant delays in accessing medical care as well as increased usage of emergency services for primary care needs. The lack of preventative services and reliable primary care availability led to increased hospitalizations, decreased quality of care, and increased cost of care. Many programs have sought to address this issue by implementing the practice of home visits into medical education and practice. Several of these programs along with 12 home-based care programs participated in a 5-year Medicare demonstration project called "Independence at Home." The results of this project found that providing 24/7 access to team coordinated care in addition to guaranteed 48 hour post-emergency department (ED)/hospital follow-up appointments with a primary care provider, resulted in savings upward of $33 million in health care cost.[33]

Although these trends in medicine are encouraging, there is still a long way to go in improving access to health care in the Unites States. With the ever-changing political climate, continued funding for community health centers is tentative at best. Although the need for home base care is clear and economically favorable, only a small percentage of primary physicians currently offer home care services.[33]

Despite boasting the highest per capita health care spending, the United States is still much less efficient than other developed countries in ensuring adequate health care for its residents.[23] Therefore, it is imperative for physicians and public officials to continue to advocate for improvements in access to primary care to ensure favorable patient outcomes and reduce health disparities.

The Role of the PCP in the Context of a Larger Health Care System in Addressing Health Inequity

Improvements in health inequity and providing greater access to high quality care for individuals who are disproportionately adversely affected by social determinants of health can be achieved in the sphere of primary care when structural and clinical solutions are made available for implementation by the primary care physician.

At a structural level, the National Academies of Sciences, Engineering and Medicine released their report in 2021 outlining the five necessary objectives which must be met to implement high-quality primary care that improves inequity in health care: (1) pay for primary care teams to care for people, not physicians to deliver services; (2) ensure that high-quality primary care is available to every individual and family in every community; (3) train primary care teams were people live and work; (4) design information technology that serves patient, their families, and the interprofessional primary care team; and (5) ensure that high-quality primary care is implemented.[34]

Conversely, screening for social and behavioral determinants of health, understanding the importance of trauma, and recognizing cultural racial and other defining characteristics of the patients served, and then building clinical operations, such as the utilization of team-based approaches to care and the leveraging of population-based tools found in modern electronic health records, are solutions that the primary care provider (PCP) can implement at the clinical level.[35–37]

Barbara Starfield's 4 Cs of primary care: first contact, continuity of care, coordination of care, and comprehensiveness are widely recognized as the key elements in developing a successful primary care model which can improve health outcomes.[38]

It has recently been proposed that these four elements of primary care, though, may not be enough to address the needs of vulnerable and underserved populations. Those facing enhanced social barriers to care require additional considerations from their primary care provider, an additional 5 Cs: convenience, cultural humility, structural competency, community engagement, and collaboration.[39]

These themes of payment reform, universal access to care, health care workforce that resembles the diversity of the patient population, innovations in health care information technology (IT), and patient-centered strategies that embrace high-quality care are frequently referenced in discussions related to improving primary care and health inequities.

The American Academy of Family Physicians has created the EveryONE Project Toolkit, an online resource designed to help the primary care physician working with underserved and vulnerable population.

The EveryONE toolkit deals with four specific areas of practice transformation and advocacy (1) implicit bias training—ways to help the care team understand unconscious bias and give them the tools they need to reduce the negative impact on patients; (2) leadership for health equity—how to create an intentional focus on health equity for patients and ways to implement team-based approaches to SDoH; (3) assessment and action—screening tools to better understand patients' social needs and help identify available resources; and (4) community collaboration and advocacy—understanding the role of the physician advocate.[40]

The primary care physician's understanding of disease and social inequity along with her standing in the community, and her professional access and opportunities makes her well suited to advocate for such structural change—expanding Medicaid, legislation improving payment and access to health insurance coverage, advocating for social change through professional associations, hospital, and hospital system associations, by building relationships with elected officials or by becoming an elected official and through community partnerships and education of community groups. Promoting and reinforcing public health messaging and advocating for social justice and greater health equity in various venues, including academic and media opportunities, are all tools at the disposal of the physician advocate.[41]

CASE STUDY

Part 3: Outcome

The patient was able to keep her follow-up appointment and her PCP identifies that she has lost a whopping 14 pounds. Her mammogram and FIT tests were all normal. The patient's repeat PHQ 9 has significantly improved but she still has depression. The patient's blood sugar is normal and her A1c is now 5.6. The patient reports that her back pain has resolved with the weight loss and back exercises. The patient reports that she has qualified for Medicaid and is now willing to take medication for her depression.

On her 2 week follow-up call with the nurse, the patient denies any side effects from the medication. At her 6 week follow-up with her PCP, the patient reports she feels much better and reports that her depression has greatly improved.

CLINICS CARE POINTS

- Five key objectives have been determined to be necessary to develop equity in health care:
  1. Payment reform—pay for primary care teams to take care of people.
  2. Ensure high-quality primary care is available to all people.
  3. Primary care teams should draw from the communities they serve.
  4. Information technology should be leveraged appropriately.
  5. Clinical deliver of high-quality primary care is necessary.
- The American Academy of Family Physicians has developed the EveryONE Toolkit, which is an on-line resource designed to help the PCP accomplish practice transformation and develop advocacy tools to benefit vulnerable populations.

REFERENCES

1. Center for the Study of Social Policy (CSSP). Key Equity Terms & Concepts: A Glossary for Shared Understanding, 2019. Available at: https://cssp.org/wp-content/uploads/2019/09/Key-Equity-Terms-and-Concepts-vol1.pdf. Accessed March 22, 2023.
2. Centers for Disease Control and Prevention. What is Health Equity? Available at: https://www.cdc.gov/healthequity/whatis/index.html. Accessed March 26, 2023.

3. World Health Organization. Health Inequality Monitor. Available at: https://www.who.int/data/inequality-monitor/about#:~:text=Health%20equity%20is%20the%20absence,economic%2C%20demographic%20or%20geographic%20characteristics. Accessed March 28, 2023.
4. The Commonwealth Fund. Achieving Racial and Ethnic Equity in U.S. Health Care. Available at: https://www.commonwealthfund.org/publications/scorecard/2021/nov/achieving-racial-ethnic-equity-us-health-care-state-performance. Accessed March 20, 2023.
5. Hill L, Ngudda N, Artiga S. Kaiser Family Foundation. Key Data on Health and Health Care by Race and Ethnicity. Available at: https://www.kff.org/racial-equity-and-health-policy/report/key-data-on-health-and-health-care-by-race-and-ethnicity/. Accessed March 03, 2023.
6. Weinstein JN, Geller A and Negussie Y, Baciu. In: National Academies of Sciences, Engineering, and Medicine. 2017. Communities in Action: Pathways to Health Equity, The National Academies Press; Washington, DC, 101.
7. Centers for Control and Prevention. Impact of Racism on our Nation's Health. Available at: https://www.cdc.gov/minorityhealth/racism-disparities/impact-of-racism.html. Accessed March 10, 2023.
8. Prüss-Üstün A, Wo lf J, Corvalán C, et al. Preventing disease through healthy environments: a global assessment of the burden of disease from environmental risks. World Health Organization; 2016.
9. Radley DC, Collins, SR. Baumgartner, JC. 2020 Scorecard on State Health System Performance. The Commonwealth Fund. Available at: https://2020scorecard.commonwealthfund.org/files/Radley_State_Scorecard_2020.pdf. Accessed March 22, 2023.
10. Blumenthal D, Mort E, Edwards J. The efficacy of primary care for vulnerable population groups. Health Serv Res 1995;30(1 Pt 2):253.
11. Belle D, Doucet J. Poverty, inequality, and discrimination as sources of depression among US women. Psychol Women Q 2003;27(2):101–13.
12. Singh GK, Siahpush M. Widening socioeconomic inequalities in US life expectancy, 1980–2000. Int J Epidemiol 2006;35(4):969–79.
13. Khullar D, Chokshi DA. Health, income, & poverty: Where we are & what could help. Health Aff 2018;10(10):1377.
14. Short SE, Zacher M. Women's Health: Population Patterns and Social Determinants. Annu Rev Sociol 2022;48:277–98.
15. Centers for Disease Control and Prevention. Lesbian, Gay, Bisexual, and Transgender Health. LGBTQ+ Youth. Available at: https://www.cdc.gov/lgbthealth/youth.htm. Accessed March 02, 2023.
16. Mayer KH, Bradford JB, Makadon HJ, et al. Sexual and gender minority health: what we know and what needs to be done. Am J Publ Health 2008 Jun;98(6):989–95.
17. Centers for Disease Control and Prevention. Rural Health. Available at: https://www.cdc.gov/ruralhealth/about.html. Accessed March 04, 2023.
18. Okoro CA, Hollis ND, Cyrus AC, et al. Prevalence of disabilities and health care access by disability status and type among adults—United States, 2016. MMWR Morb Mortal Wkly Rep 2018 Aug 8;67(32):882.
19. Mather M, Jacobsen LA, Pollard KM. Aging in the United States. Population Bulletin 2015;70(2).
20. Funk M, Drew N, Freeman M, Faydi E. Mental health and development: targeting people with mental health conditions as a vulnerable group. World Health Organization; 2010.

21. Agency for Healthcare Research and Quality. Topic: Access to Healthcare. Available at: https://www.ahrq.gov/topics/access-care.html#:~:text=Topic%3A%20Access%20to%20Care,into%20the%20health%20care%20system. Accessed April 04, 2023.
22. Shi L. The impact of primary care: a focused review. Scientifica 2012;2012: 432892.
23. Starfield B, Shi L. Policy relevant determinants of health: an international perspective. Health Pol 2002;60(3):201–18.
24. Allen EM, Call KT, Beebe TJ, et al. Barriers to care and healthcare utilization among the publicly insured. Medical care 2017;55(3):207–14.
25. Fitzpatrick AL, Powe NR, Cooper LS, et al. Barriers to health care access among the elderly and who perceives them. Am J Publ Health 2004;94(10):1788–94.
26. Schneider EC, Shah A, Doty MM, et al. Reflecting poorly: health care in the US compared to other high-income countries. New York: Commonwealth Fund; 2021.
27. Lin Y, Monnette A, Shi L. Effects of Medicaid expansion on poverty disparities in health insurance coverage. Int J Equity Health 2021;20(1):1.
28. Coen-Sanchez K, Ebenso B, El-Mowafi IM, et al. Repercussions of overturning Roe v. Wade for women across systems and beyond borders. Reprod Health 2022;19(1):1–5.
29. Finegold K, Conmy A, Chu RC, et al. Trends in the US uninsured population. Washington, DC: Office of the Assistant Secretary for Planning and Evaluation; 2021.
30. Kaiser Family Foundation. State Health Facts. Status of State Action on the Medicaid Expansion Decision. Available at: https://www.kff.org/health-reform/state-indicator/state-activity-around-expanding-medicaid-under-the-affordable-care-act/?currentTimeframe=0&sortModel=%7B%22colId%22:%22Location%22,%22sort%22:%22asc%22%7D. Accessed March 28, 2023.
31. Hayes SL, Riley P, Radley DC, et al. Reducing racial and ethnic disparities in access to care: has the Affordable Care Act made a difference. Issue Brief (Public Policy Inst Am Assoc Retired Persons) 2017;2017:1–4.
32. Saloner B, Wilk AS, Levin J. Community health centers and access to care among underserved populations: a synthesis review. Med Care Res Rev 2020;77(1):3–18.
33. Warshaw R. Housecall medicine makes a comeback. AAMC News. Available at: https://www.aamc.org/news-insights/house-call-medicine-makes-comeback. Accessed 03/21/23.
34. Phillips RL, McCauley LA, Koller CF. Implementing High-Quality Primary Care: A Report From the National Academies of Sciences, Engineering, and Medicine. JAMA 2021;325(24):2437–8.
35. O'Neill B, Ferrer R, O'Brien P, et al. Improving equity through primary care: Proceedings of the 2019 Toronto international conference on quality in primary care. Ann Fam Med 2020;18(4):364–9.
36. Teutsch S, Carey TS, Pignone M. Health equity in preventive services: the role of primary care. Am Fam Physician 2020;102(5):264–5.
37. World Health Organization. The world health report 2008 : primary health care now more than ever. World Health Organization; 2008. https://apps.who.int/iris/handle/10665/43949.
38. Starfield B. Measuring the attainment of primary care. Acad Med 1979;54(5):361–9.
39. Henry TL, Britz JB, Louis JS, et al. Health equity: the only path forward for primary care. Ann Fam Med 2022;20(2):175–8.

40. American Academy of Family Physicians. The EveryONE Project Toolkit. Advancing Health Equity through Family Medicine. Available at: https://www.aafp.org/family-physician/patient-care/the-everyone-project/toolkit.html. Accessed March 14, 2023.
41. Earnest MA, Wong SL, Federico SG. Perspective: physician advocacy: what is it and how do we do it? Acad Med 2010;85(1):63–7.

Economic Determinants of Health Disparities and the Role of the Primary Care Provider

Paul D. Juarez, PhD

KEYWORDS

- Economic determinants of health • Points of care interventions • Public policy
- Health in all policy interventions

KEY POINTS

- Social and economic determinants of health contribute more to health disparities than genetics, lifestyle choices, and access to care, combined.
- Growing up in poverty and exposure to other early life stressors often does not cause immediate health consequences but significantly affects an individual's health over the life course.
- Within the health care system, there are multiple federal and state initiatives, Medicare and Medicaid-specific initiatives, and other public policies being undertaken to address social and economic determinants to improve health equity.
- Outside of the health care system, health in all policy initiatives seek to shape policies and practices in nonhealth sectors in ways to decrease disparities and promote health equity.

INTRODUCTION

Being poor is bad for your health. People of lower socioeconomic status (SES) are disproportionately negatively affected by a host of place-based, social, and economic factors, including environmental injustices, over the life course, that adversely affect their health and lead to increased rates of disease, premature death, and shortened lifespan. Typically, no single factor explains the relationship between economic factors and health. Instead, the cumulative impact of multiple, social, economic, and environmental factors from conception on, continuing over the life course, needs to be considered.[1] Cumulative social, economic, and environmental factors have both a direct and indirect impact on health, and together, have a greater impact than health care access, lifestyle choices, and genetic makeup, combined.[2]

Department of Family & Community Medicine, Meharry Medical College, 1005 Dr. DB Todd Jr. Boulevard, Nashville, TN 37208, USA
E-mail address: pjuarez@mmc.edu

Prim Care Clin Office Pract 50 (2023) 561–577
https://doi.org/10.1016/j.pop.2023.05.002

DISCUSSION

Economic determinants of health are composed of individual attributes and societal conditions in which people live, work, play, learn, and pray that shape health over the course of their lives.[3,4] Living in poverty, unsafe neighborhoods, and environmental injustice communities with limited access to health promoting resources and quality health care have both an immediate and direct impact on one's health, which result in biological changes that may not be outwardly manifested for many years.[5] Many of the external factors affecting health lie beyond the health care system in the broader social and economic systems of society.[6]

Socioeconomic conditions and other environmental stressors frequently found in low-income neighborhoods often lead to environmental injustices that contribute to poor personal health outcomes and population-level health disparities among racial, ethnic, and other socially vulnerable and medically underserved populations.[7] Environmental injustice is the inequitable and disproportionate exposure of poor, minority, and disenfranchised populations to toxic chemical and nonchemical stressors found most commonly in low-income communities.[8] Personal income, wealth, education, employment, neighborhood deprivation, as well as protective factors, and social and economic policies, interact in complex ways to affect biological mechanisms and pathways that lead to the onset and progression of disease and population-level disparities.[9] Toxic, nonchemical exposures are composed of social and economic determinants of health, found most commonly among populations by ethnicity, race, SES, and health status, and associated with higher incidence and prevalence of a range of diseases, including asthma,[10–12] obesity,[13–15] diabetes,[16] lung cancer,[17] and mental health and developmental problems.[18,19]

Social and economic drivers of health care disparities among minority communities include limited financial and social resources, neighborhood conditions, lack of green space, access to healthy food, access to quality education, old and dilapidated housing stock, and lack of access to culturally and linguistically competent health care providers.[20] Low income persons experiencing neighborhood deprivation are particularly vulnerable to the effects of stressful economic factors because they commonly have fewer personal financial resources, less effective coping strategies, and more potent sources of stress.[21–23] Examples of adverse health outcomes linked to economic factors include asthma attributed to certain home environments[24]; diabetes-related hospital admissions related to food insecurity[25,26]; falls due to physical barriers[27]; safety hazards[28] because of an absence of needed home modifications[29]; frequent use of the emergency department by persons experiencing homelessness[30,31]; and a risk of stress-related illness resulting from unemployment,[32,33] among other things.[34,35]

Growing up in poverty and exposure to early life stressors, such as adverse childhood exposures (ACEs), often do not cause immediately identifiable health consequences but they can still significantly affect an individual's health over the life course.[36,37] ACEs are traumatic events that occur before a child reaches the age of 18 years. Such experiences can interfere with a person's health, opportunities, and stability throughout his or her lifetime—and can even affect future generations.[37] ACEs, such as child abuse and neglect and witnessing domestic violence, are more commonly found among children of low compared to high SES.[38] A growing body of research suggests that ACEs can cause "lasting alterations to the endocrine, autonomic, and central nervous system" during early childhood and may have long-term effects on the body, including speeding up the processes of disease and aging and compromising immune systems."[39,40]

Adverse health outcomes and behaviors that have been found to be associated with ACEs include chronic obstructive pulmonary disease,[41] cardiometabolic disease,[42,43] depression,[44,45] fetal death,[46] early initiation of sexual activity,[47] risk for intimate partner violence,[48,49] liver disease,[50] sexually transmitted diseases,[51] unintended pregnancies,[52,53] and early mortality.[54] The WHO Mental Health Survey administered in 21 countries attributed 30% of adult mental illnesses to ACEs.[55] Another survey conducted by the WHO in 8 Eastern European countries found a strong association between ACEs, health harming behaviors, and mental health outcomes,[56] including smoking, alcohol dependence and abuse, illicit drug use, suicide attempts, violence victimization and perpetration, and overall quality of life.[57–59] A recent survey of adults conducted in 27 US states found that 16% of respondents reported having experienced 4 or more types of ACEs.[60] In addition to the personal biological effects of ACEs, social and economic conditions, such as parental wealth and neighborhood income, may affect one's ability to successfully navigate critical life stages, such as transitions from school to work, being single to marriage, and childrearing to retirement, all of which require material resources that people living in lower SES households often lack.[61]

Although ACEs are experienced by persons across all sectors of society, socially and economically vulnerable population are more likely to be exposed.[62,63] Race and ethnicity are often linked to both social and economic factors and health disparities, including racism, at both an individual and institutional level.[64–66] Since 2018, at least 37 states and the District of Columbia have enacted or adopted legislation related to ACEs, including laws that address childhood trauma, child adversity, toxic stress, and ACEs specifically. Public policies have been enacted to address ACEs include creating a new taskforce or work group, implementing training for educators and others on ACEs or trauma-informed practices, and strengthening behavioral health supports for children.

Wealth is essential for economic security and health and well-being. Wealth gives households the ability to pursue an education, take employment, move to new neighborhoods, buy a home, and start a business. Poverty, in contrast, often limits access to educational and employment opportunities, which further contribute to income inequality and perpetuate cyclical effects of poverty. The racial wealth gap in the United States is the result of lost income and lost opportunity, compounded over time, and closely tracks the history of racial discrimination (**Table 1**). Patterns of wealth accumulation and wealth mobility during working life contribute to this inequality. The racial wealth gap reflects both different wealth dynamics and different starting positions. A white person who has median wealth in their early thirties is expected to have more wealth in their late fifties than a black person who has 90th percentile wealth in their thirties. On top of having less wealth than white Americans to begin with, black Americans are both less likely to move up the economic ladder and more likely to slide down it.[67]

Populations experiencing wealth inequality tend to report poorer health outcomes[68] and insufficient money to meet basic material needs such as safe housing,[69] high quality

Table 1
Wealth gap by race/ethnicity

Wealth Gap	For Every Dollar	Average Wealth (2022)
White	$1	$1,273,000
Black	$0.25	$316,000
Latino	$0.23	$291,000

food,[70] and preventive medical services.[71,72] Wealth inequality is strongly associated with infant death,[73] teen birth rates,[74] HIV,[75,76] violence,[77,78] all causes of death,[79] and reduced social and economic opportunities.[80] In addition, residents of impoverished communities often have reduced access to resources that are needed to support a healthy quality of life, such as stable housing, healthy-eating-patterns title= "https://health.gov/healthypeople/priority-areas/social-determinants-health/literature-summaries/access-foods-support-healthy-eating-patterns,"> and access to healthy foods, and safe neighborhoods.

After centuries of racial discrimination and economic exclusion, both US racial wealth and health gaps remain stubbornly large (**Fig. 1**).[81] The racial wealth gap not only perpetuates past harms but sustains the social and economic forces that ensure the continuance of health disparities. The emerging field of exposomics research increasingly is showing how social inequalities can act across multiple biological layers, leading to physiological changes (such as body weight and blood pressure) and molecular changes (reflected by epigenetic, transcriptomic, proteomic, and metabolomic markers), leading to disease onset.[82] To address disparities in health outcomes, interventions that address broader social and economic conditions, such as systemic racism, are needed. Systemic racism has been found to directly affect underlying biological mechanisms and pathways of stress that lead to the onset and progression of poor health conditions.[83]

Neighborhood provides the social and economic contexts in which children and adults live their lives and often determines the educational, work, and economic opportunities available to them. The physical conditions of high deprivation neighborhoods pose many challenges that make healthy lifestyles difficult to achieve. People who live in neighborhoods with higher levels of deprivation are more likely to be

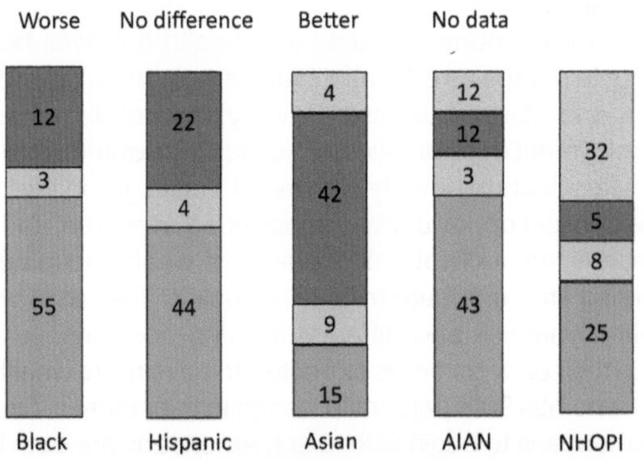

Fig. 1. Health and health care among people of color compared to white people. Number of measures for which racial/ethnic groups fared better, the same, or worse compared to white people: Note: Measures are for the most recent year for which data are available. "Better or "Worse" indicates a statistically significant difference from white people at the $P < 0.05$ level. No difference indicates no statistically significant difference. "Data limitation" indicates no separate data for a racial/ethnic group, insufficient data for a reliable estimate, or comparisons, or not possible due to overlapping samples. AIAN refers to American Indian or Alaska Native, HHOPI refers to Native Hawaiian or Other Pacific Islander. Persons of Hispanic origin may be any race but are categorized as Hispanic for this analysis: other. Groups are non-Hispanic. (*From* Hill, L, Ndugga, N, and Artiga, S. Key Data on Health and Health Care by Race and Ethnicity. Published March 15, 2023. Accessed on April 20, 2023. https://www.kff.org/racial-equity-and-health-policy/report/key-data-on-health-and-health-care-by-race-and-ethnicity/.)

non-white, and to experience poverty, overcrowding, and severe housing cost burden,[84] even after taking many common health risk factors into account, such as smoking, into account.[85] For example, persons who live in poorer neighborhoods tend to have fewer parks and recreational facilities available for physical activity compared to those who live in wealthier neighborhoods.[86,87] Likewise, people who live in high deprivation neighborhoods are more likely to live in older, poorly maintained houses with high levels of exposures to indoor pollutants, including allergens, such as chemicals, cockroaches, and dust mites, that increase the frequency and severity of asthma attacks.[88] Similarly, children who live in low-income neighborhoods are more likely to live near highways and major streets with exposure to unhealthy air pollutants, including PM2.5, PM10, ozone, nitrogen dioxide, carbon monoxide, and sulfur dioxide.[89]

INTERVENTION STRATEGIES

The US health system is a mix of public and private, for-profit and nonprofit, insurers, health care providers, and community partners. Persons who are uninsured often "fall between the health care cracks" because even though they are employed with incomes exceeding the federal poverty level, they lack the economic resources for private health care. A growing number of public and private initiatives have been proposed to address social determinants of health within and outside of the health care system to eliminate disparities and promote health equity.

Public response: The federal government provides funding for the national Medicare program for adults aged 65 years and older and some people with disabilities as well as for various programs for veterans and low-income people, including Medicaid, the Children's Health Insurance Program, and federally qualified health centers. States manage and pay for aspects of local coverage and the safety net. Private insurance, the dominant form of coverage, is provided primarily by employers.[90]

Health Resources Service Administration (HRSA). HRSA is the primary federal agency for improving health care to people who are medically underserved or live in underserved areas. HRSA has developed a system for identifying socially vulnerable and medically underserved people within a defined geographic area who have a shortage of available primary, dental, or mental health care providers (health professions shortage area [HPSA]: geographic or populations); and populations with a lack of access to primary care services (medically underserved areas [MUAs]/medically underserved populations [MUP]) (https://bhw.hrsa.gov/workforce-shortage-areas/shortage-designation. Accessed on 3/26/2023) (**Table 2**). HPSAs, on the one hand, are geographic areas, populations, or facilities that have a shortage of primary, dental, or mental health care providers. A geographic HPSA can be an area that has a shortage of providers for an entire group of people; a population HPSA has a shortage of providers for a specific group of people within a defined geographic area (eg, low-income, migrant farm workers); and a facility HPSA is a public or nonprofit private medical facility that serves a population or geographic area with a shortage of providers. MUAs, on the other hand, are geographic areas that have a shortage of primary care health services, such as a whole county, a group of neighboring counties, a group of urban census tracts, or a group of county or civil divisions. In contrast, MUPs are specific populations that have a shortage of primary care health services, defined as people who are experiencing homelessness, low-income, eligible for Medicaid, Native Americans, or identified as migrant farm workers. These populations often face economic, cultural, or language barriers to

Table 2
Socially vulnerable and underserved populations

Socially Vulnerable	Undeserved
• Have high risk for multiple health problems and/or pre-existing conditions	• Receive fewer health care services
• Have limited life options (eg, financial, educational, housing)	• Have a lack of familiarity with the health care delivery system
Display fear and distrust in accessing government programs or disclosing sensitive information about family members	• Encounter barrier to accessing primary health care services (eg, economic, cultural, and/or linguistic)
Have a limited ability to understand or give informed consent without the assistance of language services (eg, consumers with limited english proficiency [LEP] or cognitive impairments)	• Face a shortage of readily available providers
• Have mobility impairments	
• Have a lack of access to transportation services	
• Have a lowered capacity to communicate effectively	
• Face any type of discrimination	

health care and often have reduced access to resources that are needed to support a healthy quality of life, such as stable housing, healthy foods, and safe neighborhoods.[91,92]

In addition, HRSA designates and funds a national network of Federally Qualified Health Centers (FQHCs). Community health centers play a critical role in the US health care system, delivering care to over 29 million people today. By statute, community health centers must operate in or serve medically underserved communities and populations. In addition, they must prospectively adjust fees according to a schedule adjusted for family income and be governed by a board, a majority of whose members are patients of the health centers. Today, health centers represent the nation's single largest investment in comprehensive primary health care for urban and rural communities and populations designated as medically underserve, defined in terms of poverty, evidence of unmet need for primary health care, and shortages of primary health care professionals.[93] Compared to the US population overall, health center patients are nearly 5 times as likely to be poor, more than twice as likely to be uninsured, and two-and-a half times as likely to be covered by Medicaid.[93] (**Fig. 2**)[81]

Federal and state initiatives. Within the health care system, a number of waivers to both the Medicare and Medicaid programs have been approved by the Center for Medicare and Medicaid (CMS) to provide more efficient procedures for treating patients in response to the COVID pandemic. A sample of Medicare waivers is presented in **Table 3**.

Medicaid initiatives. A number of delivery and payment reform initiatives within Medicaid intend to link and include health care and social needs as part of Section 1115 Medicaid demonstration waivers. Some state Medicaid programs have launched Accountable Care Organization (ACO) models that include population-based

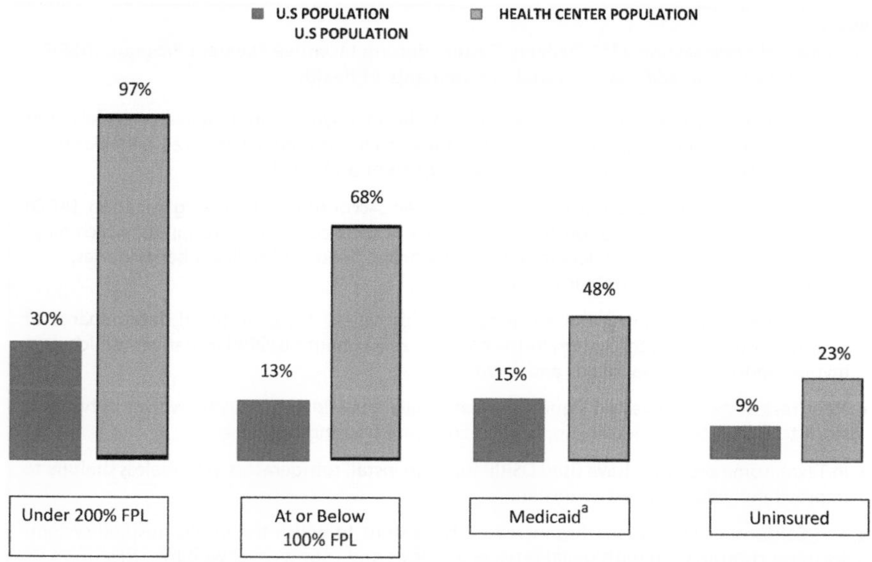

Fig. 2. Health center patients are disproportionately poor, uninsured, and publicly insured. FPL, federal poverty level. [a]Medicaid alone and not in combination with other insurance. (*Adapted from* Hill, L, Ndugga, N, and Artiga, S. Key Data on Health and Health Care by Race and Ethnicity. Published March 15, 2023. Accessed on April 20, 2023. https://www.kff.org/racial-equity-and-health-policy/report/key-data-on-health-and-health-care-by-race-and-ethnicity/.)

payments or total cost of care formulas, which provide incentives for providers to address the broad needs of Medicaid beneficiaries, including the social determinants of health. A review of strategies from approved state Medicaid 1115 waivers summarized by the Kaiser Family Foundation is presented in **Box 1**:[94]

Table 3
Medicare waivers in response to COVID-19 pandemic

Emergency Medical Treatment & Labor Act (EMTALA)	Allows hospitals, psychiatric hospitals, and critical access hospitals to screen patients at a location offsite from the hospital's campus to prevent the spread of COVID-19, as long as it is consistent with a state's emergency preparedness or pandemic plan.
CFR §482.41 and 42 CFR §485.623	Allows for increased flexibilities for surge capacity and patient quarantine at hospitals, psychiatric hospitals, and critical access hospitals (CAHs) as a result of COVID-19.
t 42 CFR §482.12(a) (8)– (9) for hospitals and §485.616(c) for CAHs	Makes it easier for telemedicine services to be furnished to the hospital's patients through an agreement with an off-site hospital. (Set to expire May 11, 2023 with the expiration of the federally declared public health emergency, unless additional legislation is passed.)
42 CFR § 485.631(b) (2).	Waives the requirement that a doctor of medicine or osteopathy be physically present to provide medical direction, consultation, and supervision for the services provided.

Box 1
Examples of state section 1115 Delivery System Reform Incentive Payment Program (DSRIP) Medicaid waivers to address the social determinants of health

- Colorado and Oregon are implementing Medicaid payment and delivery models that provide care through regional entities that focus on integration of physical, behavioral, and social services as well as community engagement and collaboration.
- Several state Medicaid programs have launched Accountable Care Organization (ACO) models that include population-based payments or total cost of care formulas, which may provide incentives for providers to address the broad needs of Medicaid beneficiaries, including the social determinants of health.
- Some state Medicaid programs are supporting providers' focus on social determinants of health through "Delivery System Reform Incentive Payment" (DSRIP) initiatives, which may involve addressing social needs and factors.
- New York state has invested significant state dollars outside of its DSRIP waiver in housing stock to ensure that a better supply of appropriate housing is available.
- In Texas, some providers have used DSRIP funds to install refrigerators in homeless shelters to improve individuals' access to insulin.
- The California DSRIP waiver has increased the extent to which the public hospital systems focus on coordination with social services agencies and county-level welfare offices.
- The Louisiana Department of Health formed a partnership with the Louisiana Housing Authority to establish a Permanent Supportive Housing (PSH) program with the dual goals of preventing and reducing homelessness and unnecessary institutionalization among people with disabilities. Louisiana's Medicaid program covers three phases of tenancy support services for Medicaid beneficiaries in permanent supportive housing: pre-tenancy services (housing search assistance, application assistance etc.), move-in services, and ongoing tenancy services.

Outside of the health care system. Outside of the health care system, an array of initiatives have sought to address the needs of poor and medically underserved populations, both at the clinical point of care and through shaping policies and practices in nonhealth sectors in ways that promote health and health equity.[91,92]

Point of care. Primary care providers can provide an important means to mitigating threats to individual and community health posed by adverse conditions by addressing social and economic determinants of health (SEDH). There are both patient-specific and clinic-based interventions that primary care providers can undertake to address SEDH at the point of care. Although there is not currently a recommended evidence base of social determinants of health to collect or how to collect them, the Institute of Medicine (IOM)[95] has identified 17 social, economic, and behavioral domains for consideration to incorporate into all electronic health record (EHRs), including race/ethnicity, education, financial resource strain, stress, depression, physical activity, tobacco use and exposure, alcohol use, social connections and social isolation, exposure to violence: intimate partner violence, and neighborhood and community compositional characteristics.[95] Gold and colleagues[96] support using the institute of medicine (IOM) recommended domains, modified to address local context. A suggested list of point of care interventions for primary care providers to address SEDH is presented in the Clinics Care Points at the end of this article.

Policies and practices in nonhealth sectors Policies also have been implemented across public, non-health care domains and in partnership with private partners to address the direct and indirect impacts on health and health equity. A "Health in All Policies" approach incorporates health considerations into decision making across sectors and policy areas[97,98] (**Fig. 3**).[99] A Health in All Policies approach identifies the ways in which decisions in multiple sectors affect health, and how improved health can support the goals of these multiple sectors. It engages diverse partners and stakeholders to work together to promote health, equity, and sustainability, while simultaneously advancing other goals such as promoting job creation and economic stability, transportation access and mobility, a strong agricultural system, and improved educational attainment.

A Health in All Policies approach has been used to respond to health issues across a wide array of public agencies and in collaboration with private partners to increase availability and accessibility of public transportation for persons to commute to their jobs, provide access to affordable healthy food and health care, and to address other important drivers of health and wellness. States and localities are utilizing the Health in All Policies approach by employing task forces and workgroups focused on bringing together leaders across agencies and the community to collaborate and focus on health and health equity.[100] At the federal level, the Affordable Care Act (ACA) established the National Prevention Council, which brings together senior leadership from 20 federal departments, agencies, and offices, who worked with the Prevention Advisory Group, stakeholders, and the general public to develop the National Prevention Strategy.[101] At the local level, nutrition programs and policies have been used not only to support healthy diet and nutrition for low income children and families, but to increase the production and consumption of healthy foods, support patronage at healthier corner stores in low-income communities, and fund the start-up of farm to school programs[94] and community and school gardens[97] (**Box 2**). Early childhood education programs have been targeted to children in low-income families and communities of color to reduce achievement gaps, improve the health of low-income students, and promote health equity[98]

Conclusion: There continues to be growing recognition of the relationship between neighborhoods and health, with zip code understood to be a stronger predictor of a person's health than their genetic code.[102] A number of initiatives now focus on implementing coordinated strategies across different sectors in neighborhoods with social, economic, and environmental barriers that lead to poor health outcomes and health disparities. Place-based initiatives have focused on implementing cross-sector

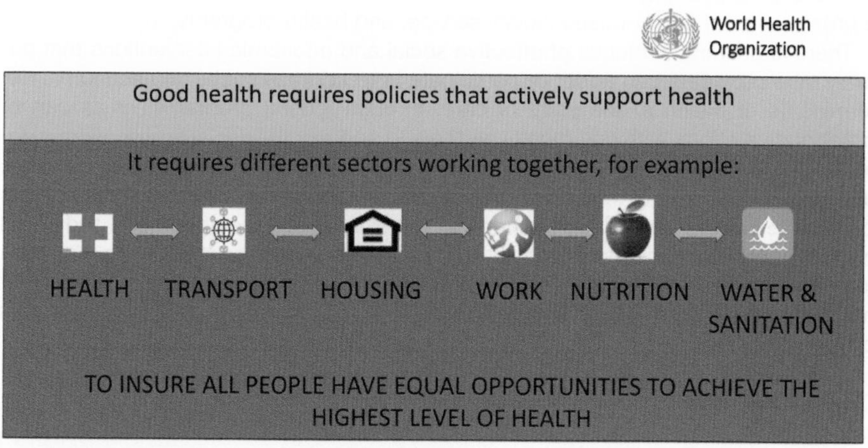

Fig. 3. What is health in all policies? (*Adapted from* World Health Organization. https://twitter.com/WHO/status/570499107116216320.)

Box 2
Public policy strategies to promote health equity in non-health care sector

- Home visiting programs improve parenting skills and the home environment, reduce unintentional injury, enhance maternal employment and education, and improve intellectual development among children.
- Healthy places include transforming communities by encouraging mixed land use; providing good public transportation and pedestrian and bicycle infrastructure; containing affordable housing, green space, parks and community centers; and creating outlets for fresh fruits and vegetables.
- Community Transformation recommends direct community-based interventions and policy approaches for reducing the impact of SES on health. Community Transformation focuses on reducing health disparities and provides strategies that increase physical activity, improve nutrition, reduce smoking, and assure quality medical care. These approaches together might particularly benefit persons experiencing neighborhood deprivation who often face challenges in securing resources that promote health.
- Federal Department of Health and Human Services National Partnership for Action to End Health Disparities and its companion National Stakeholders Strategy for Achieving Health Equity.
- Tackling Health Inequities Through Public Health Practice. This publication offers a starting point to address fundamental causes of health inequities. It provides general approaches illustrated by specific examples for: shifting consciousness and paradigms about determinants of health.
- Studying existing policies—social, economic, educational, urban and rural development, housing, transportation, and health care financing and delivery—of other high-income countries and considering their application in the United States. Both documents suggest that policies aimed at reducing high economic inequality and paying more attention to early impact of different socio-economic variables on the lifestyle factors, like lack of physical activity, diet rich in meat, and smoking.

strategies to improve health in neighborhoods or communities with poor health outcomes.[103] For example, the Harlem Children's Zone (HCZ) project has focused on children within a 100-block area in Central Harlem with high rates of chronic disease and infant mortality as well as high rates of poverty and unemployment.[104] HCZ sought to improve the educational, economic, and health outcomes of the community through a broad range of family-based, social service, and health programs.

There is growing evidence of effective social and economic interventions that primary care providers can adopt or participate in to address social and economic determinants of health at the point of care, through federal programs, or as part of collaborative efforts with community partners to address the social and economic determinants of health. Primary care providers can write prescriptions for diet, exercise, and stress reduction; extend their office hours; collaborate with community partners; participate in team-based approaches that target individual, neighborhood and social and economic level drivers of health and disparities; and engage in advocacy activities to promote activities that promote health equity, whether through the HC system or not. Just as economic determinants of health disparities are multiple, so too must be the solutions.

CLINICS CARE POINTS

- Collect patient SEDH via multiple routes (patient surveys, direct patient data entry, practice advisories, health maintenance advisories, etc.).

- Create an SEDH data summary tab in the EHR that is automatically populated with data from any of the SDH data entry options and from SEDH-related data elsewhere in the EHR.
- Screen for structural inequities that may be affecting patient health, such as income, housing, education, employment, and neighborhood.
- Maintain a resource director of community assets for referring patients who may be experiencing economic challenges, such as prescription assistance for low-income patients, food banks, Supplemental nutrition Assistance Program (SNAP), child support, transportation, housing agencies, and disaster-related emergency assistance.
- Provide training for front-line health providers on how to screen for patient SEDH.
- Partner with outside specialized agencies, such as food banks, Family Assistance Service Centers, housing programs, community health centers, etc.
- Engage community health workers who are from similar socioeconomic and cultural backgrounds to help individual patients navigate health and economic needs and services.
- Fund embedded social service specialists in the clinic or establish partnership with community organizations.

DISCLOSURE

The author had nothing to disclose.

REFERENCES

1. Juarez PD, Matthews-Juarez P, Hood DB, et al. The public health exposome: a population-based, exposure science approach to health disparities research. Int J Environ Res Public Health 2014;11(12):12866–95.
2. Solomon GM, Morello-Frosch R, Zeise L, et al. Cumulative Environmental Impacts: Science and Policy to Protect Communities. Annu Rev Publ Health 2016;37(1):83–96.
3. Warnecke RB, Oh A, Breen N, et al. Approaching health disparities from a population perspective: the National Institutes of Health Centers for Population Health and Health Disparities. Am J Public Health 2008;98(9):1608–15.
4. Lawrence D, Graber JE, Mills SL, et al. Smoking cessation interventions in U.S. racial/ethnic minority populations: an assessment of the literature☆. Prev Med 2003;36(2):204–16.
5. Senier L, Brown P, Shostak S, et al. The Socio-Exposome: Advancing Exposure Science and Environmental Justice in a Post-Genomic Era. Environ Sociol 2017;3(2):107–21.
6. Brody JG, Morello-Frosch R, Zota A, et al. Linking exposure assessment science with policy objectives for environmental justice and breast cancer advocacy: The Northern California Household Exposure Study. Am J Publ Health 2009;99(S3):S600–9.
7. Kendzor DE, Businelle MS, Mazas CA, et al. Pathways between socioeconomic status and modifiable risk factors among African American smokers. J Behav Med 2009;32:545–57.
8. Periot M, Dron J, Austruy A, et al. Advancing Exposome Understanding and Environmental Justice Knowledge in a Major European Industrial Harbor (Fos-Sur-Mer, France) Through Longitudinal and Strongly Participatory. Research 2022. https://doi.org/10.2139/ssrn.4158292.

9. Woolf SH, Braveman P. Where health disparities begin: the role of social and economic determinants—and why current policies may make matters worse. Health affairs 2011;30(10):1852–9.
10. Cook Q, Argenio K, Lovinsky-Desir S. The impact of environmental injustice and social determinants of health on the role of air pollution in asthma and allergic disease in the United States. J Allergy Clin Immunol 2021;148(5):1089–101, e1085.
11. Harris KM. Mapping inequality: Childhood asthma and environmental injustice, a case study of St. Louis, Missouri. Social science & medicine 2019;230:91–110.
12. Lowe AA, Bender B, Liu AH, et al. Environmental concerns for children with asthma on the Navajo Nation. Annals of the American Thoracic Society 2018; 15(6):745–53.
13. Nogueira H, Gama A, Mourao I, et al. The associations of SES, obesity, sport activity, and perceived neighborhood environments: is there a model of environmental injustice penalizing Portuguese children? Am J Hum Biol 2013;25(3): 434–6.
14. Taylor WC, Hepworth JT, Lees E, et al. Obesity, Physical Activity, and the Environment: Is There a Legal Basis for Environmental Injustices? Environ Justice 2008;1(1):45–8.
15. Cureton S., Environmental victims: environmental injustice issues that threaten the health of children living in poverty, 2011, 141–147. https://doi.org/10.1515/reveh.2011.021.
16. Rosen LD, Imus D. Environmental injustice: Children's health disparities and the role of the environment. Explore 2007;3(5):524–8.
17. Mathiarasan S, Hüls A. Impact of environmental injustice on children's health—interaction between air pollution and socioeconomic status. Int J Environ Res Publ Health 2021;18(2):795.
18. Hoff MD, Rogge ME. Everything that rises must converge: Developing a social work response to environmental injustice. J Prog Hum Serv 1996;7(1):41–57.
19. Malin SA. Depressed democracy, environmental injustice: Exploring the negative mental health implications of unconventional oil and gas production in the United States. Energy Res Social Sci 2020;70:101720.
20. Siqueira CE, Gaydos M, Monforton C, et al. Effects of social, economic, and labor policies on occupational health disparities. Am J Ind Med 2014;57(5): 557–72.
21. Larson NI, Story MT, Nelson MC. Neighborhood environments: disparities in access to healthy foods in the US. Am J Prev Med 2009;36(1):74–81, e10.
22. Ingraham NE, Purcell LN, Karam BS, et al. Racial and ethnic disparities in hospital admissions from COVID-19: determining the impact of neighborhood deprivation and primary language. J Gen Intern Med 2021;36(11):3462–70.
23. Hilmers A, Hilmers DC, Dave J. Neighborhood disparities in access to healthy foods and their effects on environmental justice. Am J Publ Health 2012; 102(9):1644–54.
24. Morgan WJ, Crain EF, Gruchalla RS, et al. Results of a home-based environmental intervention among urban children with asthma. N Engl J Med 2004; 351(11):1068–80.
25. Essien UR, Shahid NN, Berkowitz SA. Food insecurity and diabetes in developed societies. Curr Diabetes Rep 2016;16:1–8.
26. Flint KL, Davis GM, Umpierrez GE. Emerging trends and the clinical impact of food insecurity in patients with diabetes. J Diabetes 2020;12(3):187–96.

27. Fernandes JB, Fernandes SB, Almeida AS, et al. Older adults' perceived barriers to participation in a falls prevention strategy. J Personalized Med 2021;11(6):450.
28. Biswas A, Harbin S, Irvin E, et al. Sex and gender differences in occupational hazard exposures: a scoping review of the recent literature. Curr Environ Health Rep 2021;1–14.
29. Bakk L, Cadet T, Lien L, et al. Home modifications among community-dwelling older adults: a closer look at race and ethnicity. J Gerontol Soc Work 2017;60(5):377–94.
30. Vohra N, Paudyal V, Price MJ. Homelessness and the use of Emergency Department as a source of healthcare: a systematic review. Int J Emerg Med 2022;15(1):1–22.
31. Salhi BA, White MH, Pitts SR, et al. Homelessness and emergency medicine: a review of the literature. Acad Emerg Med 2018;25(5):577–93.
32. Moser KA, Fox AJ, Jones D. Unemployment and mortality in the OPCS longitudinal study. Lancet 1984;324(8415):1324–9.
33. Hammarström A. Health consequences of youth unemployment—review from a gender perspective. Soc Sci Med 1994;38(5):699–709.
34. Bachrach D, Pfister H, Wallis K, et al. Addressing patients' social needs: an emerging business case for provider investment. New York, NY: Commonwealth Fund; 2014.
35. Pynoos J, Steinman BA, Do Nguyen AQ, et al. Assessing and adapting the home environment to reduce falls and meet the changing capacity of older adults. J Hous Elder 2012;26(1–3):137–55.
36. Wild CP. Complementing the genome with an "exposome": the outstanding challenge of environmental exposure measurement in molecular epidemiology. Cancer Epidemiol Biomark Prev 2005;14(8):1847–50.
37. Horsthemke B. A critical view on transgenerational epigenetic inheritance in humans. Nat Commun 2018;9(1):2973.
38. Felitti Md FVJ, Anda Md MSRF, Nordenberg Md D, et al. Relationship of Childhood Abuse and Household Dysfunction to Many of the Leading Causes of Death in Adults: The Adverse Childhood Experiences (ACE) Study. Am J Prev Med 1998;14(4):245–58.
39. Voellmin A, Winzeler K, Hug E, et al. Blunted endocrine and cardiovascular reactivity in young healthy women reporting a history of childhood adversity. Psychoneuroendocrinology 2015;51:58–67.
40. Winzeler K, Voellmin A, Hug E, et al. Adverse childhood experiences and autonomic regulation in response to acute stress: the role of the sympathetic and parasympathetic nervous systems. Hist Philos Logic 2017;30(2):145–54.
41. Anda RF, Brown DW, Dube SR, et al. Adverse childhood experiences and chronic obstructive pulmonary disease in adults. Am J Prev Med 2008;34(5):396–403.
42. Deighton S, Neville A, Pusch D, et al. Biomarkers of adverse childhood experiences: A scoping review. Psychiatr Res 2018;269:719–32.
43. Wickrama KK, O'Neal CW, Lee TK, et al. Early socioeconomic adversity, youth positive development, and young adults' cardio-metabolic disease risk. Health Psychol 2015;34(9):905.
44. Chapman DP, Whitfield CL, Felitti VJ, et al. Adverse childhood experiences and the risk of depressive disorders in adulthood. J Affect Disord 2004;82(2):217–25.

45. Lee HY, Kim I, Nam S, et al. Adverse childhood experiences and the associations with depression and anxiety in adolescents. Child Youth Serv Rev 2020; 111:104850.
46. Hillis SD, Anda RF, Dube SR, et al. The association between adverse childhood experiences and adolescent pregnancy, long-term psychosocial consequences, and fetal death. Pediatrics 2004;113(2):320–7.
47. Song W, Qian X. Adverse Childhood Experiences and Teen Sexual Behaviors: The Role of Self-Regulation and School-Related Factors. J Sch Health 2020; 90(11):830–41.
48. Mair C, Cunradi CB, Todd M. Adverse childhood experiences and intimate partner violence: Testing psychosocial mediational pathways among couples. Ann Epidemiol 2012;22(12):832–9.
49. Li Y, Herbell K, Bloom T, et al. Adverse childhood experiences and mental health among women experiencing intimate partner violence. Issues Ment Health Nurs 2020;41(9):785–91.
50. Dong M, Dube SR, Felitti VJ, et al. Adverse childhood experiences and self-reported liver disease: new insights into the causal pathway. Arch Intern Med 2003;163(16):1949–56.
51. Hillis SD, Anda RF, Felitti VJ, et al. Adverse childhood experiences and sexually transmitted diseases in men and women: a retrospective study. Pediatrics 2000; 106(1):e11.
52. Young-Wolff KC, Wei J, Varnado N, et al. Adverse childhood experiences and pregnancy intentions among pregnant women seeking prenatal care. Wom Health Issues 2021;31(2):100–6.
53. Dietz PM, Spitz AM, Anda RF, et al. Unintended pregnancy among adult women exposed to abuse or household dysfunction during their childhood. JAMA 1999; 282(14):1359–64.
54. Hughes K, Bellis MA, Hardcastle KA, et al. The effect of multiple adverse childhood experiences on health: a systematic review and meta-analysis. Lancet Public Health 2017;2(8):e356–66.
55. Kessler RC, McLaughlin KA, Green JG, et al. Childhood adversities and adult psychopathology in the WHO World Mental Health Surveys. Br J Psychiatry 2010;197(5):378–85.
56. Bellis MA, Hughes K, Leckenby N, et al. Adverse childhood experiences and associations with health-harming behaviours in young adults: surveys in eight eastern European countries. Bull World Health Organ 2014;92(9):641–55.
57. Chanlongbutra A, Singh GK, Mueller CD. Adverse Childhood Experiences, Health-Related Quality of Life, and Chronic Disease Risks in Rural Areas of the United States. J Environ Public Healt 2018;2018:7151297.
58. Vederhus JK, Timko C, Haugland SH. Adverse childhood experiences and impact on quality of life in adulthood: development and validation of a short difficult childhood questionnaire in a large population-based health survey. Qual Life Res 2021;30(6):1769–78.
59. Jia H, Lubetkin EI. Impact of adverse childhood experiences on quality-adjusted life expectancy in the U.S. population. Child Abuse Negl 2020;102:104418.
60. Merrick MT, Ford DC, Ports KA, et al. Vital signs: Estimated proportion of adult health problems attributable to adverse childhood experiences and implications for prevention—25 States, 2015–2017. Morb Mortal Wkly Rep 2019;68(44):999.
61. Sandstrom H, Huerta S. The Negtive effects of instability on child development: a research Sysnthesis. 2013.

62. Maguire-Jack K, Lanier P, Lombardi B. Investigating racial differences in clusters of adverse childhood experiences. Am J Orthopsychiatry 2020;90(1):106.
63. Liu SR, Kia-Keating M, Nylund-Gibson K, et al. Co-occurring youth profiles of adverse childhood experiences and protective factors: Associations with health, resilience, and racial disparities. Am J Community Psychol 2020;65(1–2): 173–86.
64. Elias A, Paradies Y. The costs of institutional racism and its ethical implications for healthcare. J bioeth Inq 2021;18:45–58.
65. Needham BL, Ali T, Allgood KL, et al. Institutional racism and health: A framework for conceptualization, measurement, and analysis. J Rac Ethnic Health Disp 2022;1–23.
66. Peek ME, Odoms-Young A, Quinn MT, et al. Racism in healthcare: Its relationship to shared decision-making and health disparities: A response to Bradby. Soc Sci Med 2010;71(1):13.
67. Gelrud Shire A., Pulliam C., Sabelhaus J., Smith E., Studck on the Ladder:Intragenerational wealth mobility in the United States. Future of the Middle Class Initiative. Brookins Insitute. 2022. Available at: brookings.edu/wp-content/uploads/2022/06/2022_FMCI_Intragenerational WealthMobility_Final.pdf. Accessed June 29, 2022.
68. Brown ER. Income inequalities and health disparities. West J Med 2000; 172(1):25.
69. Sengoelge M, Hasselberg M, Ormandy D, et al. Housing, income inequality and child injury mortality in E urope: a cross-sectional study. Child Care Health Dev 2014;40(2):283–91.
70. Ricciuto LE, Tarasuk VS. An examination of income-related disparities in the nutritional quality of food selections among Canadian households from 1986–2001. Soc Sci Med 2007;64(1):186–98.
71. Dickman SL, Himmelstein DU, Woolhandler S. Inequality and the health-care system in the USA. Lancet 2017;389(10077):1431–41.
72. Shi L, Starfield B, Kennedy B, et al. Income inequality, primary care, and health indicators. J Fam Pract 1999;48(4):275–84.
73. Pabayo R, Cook DM, Harling G, et al. State-level income inequality and mortality among infants born in the United States 2007–2010: A Cohort Study. BMC Public Health 2019;19(1):1333.
74. Hunter L. US teen birth rate correlates with state income inequality. Population Reference Bureau. Available at: prb.org/resources/u-s-teen-birth-rate-correlates-with-state-income-inequality/. Accessed June 2, 2023.
75. Ransome Y, Kawachi I, Braunstein S, et al. Structural inequalities drive late HIV diagnosis: the role of black racial concentration, income inequality, socioeconomic deprivation, and HIV testing. Health Place 2016;42:148–58.
76. Holmqvist G., HIV and Income Inequality: If ther is a link, what does it tell use. Working Paper number 54, April 2009. Internatioanl Policy Centre for Inclusive Growth. Available at: ipc.undp.org/IPCWorkingPaper54.pdf. Accessed June 1, 2023.
77. Kennedy BP, Kawachi I, Prothrow-Stith D, et al. Social capital, income inequality, and firearm violent crime. Soc Sci Med 1998;47(1):7–17.
78. Pabayo R, Molnar BE, Kawachi I. The role of neighborhood income inequality in adolescent aggression and violence. J Adolesc Health 2014;55(4):571–9.
79. Brodish PH, Massing M, Tyroler HA. Income inequality and all-cause mortality in the 100 counties of North Carolina. Southern Medical j-Birmingham Alabama 2000;93(4):386–91.

80. Nowatzki NR. Wealth inequality and health: a political economy perspective. Int J Health Serv 2012;42(3):403–24.
81. Hill L., Ndugga N., Artiga S., Key Data on Health and Health Care by Race and Ethnicity. Kaiser Family Foundation. Available at: kff.org/racial-equity-policy/report/key-data-on-health-and-health-care-by-race-and-ethnicity/. Accessed March 15, 2023.
82. Juarez PD, Matthews-Juarez P, Hood DI W, et al. The Public Health Exposome: A Population-based, Exposure Science Approach to Health Disparities Research. Int J Environ Res Public Health 2014;11(12):12866–95.
83. Calvin R, Winters K, Wyatt SB, et al. Racism and cardiovascular disease in African Americans. Am J Med Sci 2003;325(6):315–31.
84. Chamberlain AM, Finney Rutten LJ, Wilson PM, et al. Neighborhood socioeconomic disadvantage is associated with multimorbidity in a geographically-defined community. BMC Public Health 2020;20(1):13.
85. Townsend M.S., Obesit in low-income communities: prevalence, effects, a place to begin. J Am Diet Assoc, 106(1), 2021, 34-37.
86. Schneider S, D'Agostino A, Weyers S, et al. Facilities - No Support for the Deprivation Amplification Hypothesis. J Phys Act Health 2015;12(7):990–7.
87. Huang J-H, Hipp JA, Marquet O, et al. Neighborhood characteristics associated with park use and park-based physical activity among children in low-income diverse neighborhoods in New York City. Prev Med 2020;131:105948.
88. Simons E, Dell SD, Moineddin R, et al. Neighborhood material deprivation is associated with childhood asthma development: analysis of prospective administrative data. Can Respir J J Can Thorac Soc 2019;2019.
89. Gunier RB, Hertz A, Von Behren J, et al. Traffic density in California: socioeconomic and ethnic differences among potentially exposed children. J Expo Sci Environ Epidemiol 2003;13(3):240–6.
90. Tikkanen R, Osborn R, Mossialos E, et al. International profiles of health care systems. Commonwealth Fund 2020.
91. Kranz S, Mitchell DC, Smiciklas-Wright H, et al. Consumption of recommended food groups among children from medically underserved communities. J Am Diet Assoc 2009;109(4):702–7.
92. Redlener I. Overcoming barriers to health care access for medically underserved children. J Ambulatory Care Management 1993;16(1):21–8.
93. Shin P, Rosenbaum SJ, Paradise J. Community health centers: The challenge of growing to meet the need for primary care in medically underserved communities. 2012.
94. Henery J. Medicaid waiver tracker: approved and pending Section 1115 Waivers by state. San Francisco (CA): Kaiser Family Foundation (KFF); 2019.
95. Social IOM Capturing. Behavioral Domains in Electronic Health Records: Phase 1. Edited by Records CotRSaBDaMfEH Washington DC: Institute of Medicine, 2014.
96. Gold R, Cottrell E, Bunce A, et al. Developing Electronic Health Record (EHR) Strategies Related to Health Center Patients' Social Determinants of Health. J Am Board Fam Med 2017;30(4):428–47.
97. Puska P. Health in all policies. Eur J Publ Health 2007;17(4):328.
98. Ollila E. Health in all policies: from rhetoric to action. Scand J Publ Health 2011; 39(6_suppl):11–8.
99. National Association of Community Health Centers. 2020. Community Health Center Chartbook. Available at: nachc.org/research-and-data/research-fact-

sheets-and-infographics/2021-community-health-center-chartbook/ Figure 1-82020. Accessed April 3, 2023.
100. Hall RL, Jacobson PD. Examining whether the health-in-all-policies approach promotes health equity. Health Aff 2018;37(3):364–70.
101. Chait N, Glied S. Promoting Prevention Under the Affordable Care Act. Annu Rev Publ Health 2018;39(1):507–24.
102. Brook RD, Rajagopalan S, Pope CA, et al. Particulate matter air pollution and cardiovascular disease: an update to the scientific statement from the American heart association. Circulation 2010;121.
103. Dankwa-Mullan I, Pérez-Stable EJ. Addressing health disparities is a place-based issue106. American Public Health Association; 2016. p. 637–9.
104. McCarthy K, Jean-Louis B. Harlem children's zone. Washington, DC: Center for the Study of Social Policy; 2016.

Educational Attainment and Educational Contexts as Social Determinants of Health

Sarah V. Suiter, PhD, MS[a,*], Meredith L. Meadows, MS[a]

KEYWORDS

• Educational attainment • School context • School climate
• Social determinants of health • Health outcomes

KEY POINTS

- Education is considered a social determinant of health because access to health-promoting school environments and opportunities for educational achievement – both of which influence health – are distributed unequally.
- Adults with lower educational attainment report more chronic conditions, more functional limitations, and worse overall health; Adult educational attainment also influences the health of their children.
- Most school-aged children spend a substantial portion of their time at school. The physical environment of schools, school climate, school composition, school-based health programming, and policies all affect child health.
- Inequalities among and within schools, which are often driven by broader inequities in race, class, ability, and geographic location, influence school factors and have the potential to exacerbate and amplify existing health disparities.
- Primary care providers can affect education-related health disparities by improving their knowledge of education as a social determinant of health, participating in school-health partnerships, and advocating for equitable access to high-quality education for all.

INTRODUCTION

In 2018, Case and colleagues published a study in the Proceedings of the National Academy of Sciences exploring the effect of earning a bachelor's degree on life expectancy.[1] The researchers analyzed almost 50 million death certificates from 1990 to 2018 and calculated how many years a person who was 25 year old could expect to live between that time and age 75. This widely cited study demonstrated that people without a bachelor's degree could expect to die about 3 years earlier than those with a

[a] Department of Human & Organizational Development, Vanderbilt University, 230 Appleton Place, Peabody #90, Nashville, TN 37212, USA
* Corresponding author.
E-mail address: Sarah.v.suiter@vanderbilt.edu

Prim Care Clin Office Pract 50 (2023) 579–589
https://doi.org/10.1016/j.pop.2023.04.007 primarycare.theclinics.com
0095-4543/23/

bachelor's degree. Furthermore, they demonstrated that while the life expectancy of all Americans was rising (at the time), the life expectancy of those without a bachelor's degree was declining. The authors speculated that this difference exists because "Good jobs have become increasingly rare for workers without a college diploma, many of whom have lost their jobs to globalization and automation," and for whom the costs of health care in the absence of employer-sponsored health insurance had become prohibitive.[2] The authors define "good jobs" as those in which workers earn a living wage, have access to benefits, and work in safe environments. Indeed, a large body of evidence bears out the importance of these factors to human health, morbidity, and mortality, and demonstrates one of the many pathways through which educational attainment can influence human health. Other research has demonstrated that nearly all health outcomes are patterned by the level of education.[3] Specifically, adults with lower educational attainment report more chronic conditions, more functional limitations, and worse overall health.[3] These patterns are true across social groups; however, education appears to have stronger health effects for women than men, and stronger effects for non-Hispanic whites than adults belonging to minoritized racial and ethnic groups. Furthermore, because access to opportunities for educational attainment and advancement are themselves unequal, education is considered a *social determinant* of health. In this article, we explore the relationships between educational attainment and health. We also emphasize the importance of educational contexts as determinants of health that precede educational attainment and contribute to related health outcomes.

EXISTING FRAMEWORKS FOR UNDERSTANDING EDUCATION AS A SOCIAL DETERMINANT OF HEALTH

Health outcomes are influenced by complex, multifactorial pathways. Frameworks that seek to describe the relationship between education and health outcomes often operationalize education as a "level" of education attained (eg, "completed high school") or as years of formal schooling completed. Though not encountered often in the literature, alternative operationalizations of education that may be particularly relevant to health outcomes include measures of general cognitive skills and measures of health-specific knowledge. More recent publications have noted an ongoing lack of standardization among the research that attempts to measure key constructs in the social determinants of health,[4] one result of which is an array of terminology related to education that is sometimes used interchangeably (eg, "education level" and "education status" reflect much the same concept) and sometimes even potentially misused (eg, when "education level" serves as a singular proxy for "socioeconomic status"). In frameworks that explicitly model education *as a social determinant of health*, there is a prevailing tendency to measure education as a "level" attained. In these models, educational attainment functions like a currency, with having more generally assumed to provide more "purchasing power" with regard to health-enabling goods.

Studies of the relationship between *educational attainment* and health outcomes abound in public health literature. Educational attainment is usually posited to drive three broad intermediate outcomes: knowledge, employment, and social status. Each of these intermediate outcomes, in turn, has been theoretically or empirically linked to mediators and/or moderators of health outcomes. When many such relationships are encompassed in a model, the result is a series of links through which educational attainment is expected to influence distal outcomes related to health. One example is the model created by Egerter and colleagues[5] that we refer to throughout the article as an illustrative synthesis of the theoretic and empirical work on the relationship between educational attainment and health outcomes. In the Egerter model, individual educational attainment is seen to influence knowledge in the form of health literacy and to be a mediator of activities such as the ability to manage chronic health conditions. How well individuals manage their chronic health conditions, in turn, can have substantial impacts on health outcomes. Similarly, educational attainment is often modeled as an influence on employment, which in turn moderates income. Income subsequently affects housing and neighborhood choices, stress levels, and access to quality health care, all of which are inputs or drivers of actual health outcomes. These examples of potential pathways between educational attainment and health outcomes are but two of many illustrated in Egerter and colleagues' model. Implicit in this model and others like it is an assumption that having attained more education provides more power over health outcomes.

More recent work on education as a social determinant of health has argued for the importance of expanding the definition of "education" beyond educational attainment to include schools and school contexts as more proximal determinants of health and wellbeing. Schools serve as environments in which most children ages 5 to 18 spend much of their time, and vary greatly in terms of physical conditions, resources and services that support health and health behaviors, and social-emotional climates that affect physical and mental health. These variations mean that schools can operate as sites of health promotion, prevention, and (in some cases and to a limited extent) treatment; they also mean that inequities among and within schools can create health inequalities. In this article, we discuss education as a social determinant of health in three primary ways. First, we focus on *education as currency*, which aligns with the literature on educational attainment and health. Next, we discuss *education as context*, and argue for the importance of considering school contexts as health determinants. Finally, we discuss *education as distributed good*, regarding how broader sociopolitical forces such as racism and income inequality create contexts in which educational inequities and health inequities interact and reinforce one another.

EDUCATION AS CURRENCY

In the Egerter model, educational attainment influences knowledge in the form of *health literacy*, *coping*, and *problem-solving*. These attributes are posited to influence behaviors related to diet, exercise, preventive care, and disease management, which in turn affect health outcomes.[5]

Much empirical work supports this conceptualization of the results chain linking educational attainment to health outcomes through knowledge. Greater health literacy, in particular, is often attributed to greater educational attainment and has been associated with positive health outcomes across diverse populations and contexts. Teles and Kaya, for example, found a clear, increasing gradient between levels of education and health literacy index scores among a sample of cardiovascular patients; health literacy, in turn, was a significant predictor of 14 out of 26 health outcomes within the sample.[6] Greater health literacy has also been associated with better decision-making around health, including adhering to common guidelines for preventive care such as cancer screenings and flu shots,[7,8] increased ability to take medications as prescribed,[9] and adopting more positive behaviors such as quitting tobacco.[10]

Though not explicitly modeled by Egerter and colleagues, the link between the health literacy of parents and the health outcomes of children has also been extensively studied and lends additional empirical support for the pathways described in

Egerter and colleagues's framework. For example, a positive relationship between maternal educational attainment and infant health has been noted by many independent researchers working across diverse populations and contexts and always, to the best of our knowledge, has been found to be a significant predictor of outcomes.[11] Among both infants and older children, low levels of parental education have been associated with greater likelihood of unintentional injuries and other adverse health events.[12] Findings of links between parental education and child health are especially important given the potential for poor health in childhood to persist into adolescence and adulthood.[13]

The effect of educational attainment on health outcomes through employment is slightly more complex than the pathway through knowledge but nonetheless intuitive. Educational attainment has been theoretically or empirically linked to employment outcomes, particularly those related to *income*, *employer-provided benefits*, and *working conditions.* Each of these attributes in turn influences drivers of health outcomes. The Egerter and colleagues model posits, for example, that income influences housing and neighborhood options as well as stress levels, both of which impact health and health outcomes. Working conditions also influence stress levels, moderating exposure to hazards and the amount of control and flexibility individuals have over their own work. Employer-provided benefits (eg, health insurance, paid time-off, and wellness programs) can have more direct impacts on health outcomes by, for example, facilitating access to high-quality care, allowing time-off to seek care, and eliminating the precarity and stress associated with not having these essential supports.

Research supports many of the links in the pathway between educational attainment and health outcomes through employment-related moderators as described above. In a study of Medicaid beneficiaries in Washington D.C., McCarthy[4] found a significant relationship between having at least a high school education and employment status (ie, whether an individual was employed) suggesting that individuals with education below a socially- or economically-determined threshold may in effect be rendered unemployable. It is more common for studies to control for a broader range of education levels and hence to have more generalizable findings. However, the long-term consequences of attaining little formal education are striking in this study. Clougherty and colleagues, found that *within* blue-collar and white-collar employee groups in a manufacturing firm, higher job grade was associated with a protective effect on the risk of incident hypertension after controlling for education level, income, and age.[14] The effect within blue- and white-collar groups speaks to omnipresent employment-related factors that influence health. Such factors may include an effect of job status itself, which is not included in Egerter and colleagues's framework but is posited by Clougherty and colleagues to mediate employment effects on health outcomes.[14]

Two additional studies that investigated links in the pathway between education and health outcomes through employment but with very different measurement points in the life course are Parker and colleagues and Johnson.[15,16] Parker and colleagues estimated the healthy working life expectancy (ie, the amount of time individuals are expected to remain in the workforce and in good health) of English adults aged 50+. Adults with a college degree were expected to remain healthy and working for significantly longer than those without a secondary education (11.27 years vs 7.68 years, respectively) after controlling for current health status and despite similar overall life expectancies. Thus, even if both groups were to remain in the workforce until the same age at retirement, the less educated would do so while experiencing poor health for approximately 4 years. What is perhaps more likely for the less educated workers is an earlier average retirement age, which has both individual and state-level economic consequences.

A very different type of correlational study by Johnson investigated the pathway between *childhood* educational attainment and adult health outcomes, finding, among other things, that in families in which one sibling attended Head Start (a state-funded pre-school program for low-income families) and one did not attend any pre-school, the Head Start attendee had significantly better health as an adult even after controlling for sibling fixed effects.[16] Though the mechanisms through which this occurs are not known, Johnson's results speak to cumulative effects of educational attainment in pre-adulthood and the influences these have on adult employment opportunities.

Finally, the effect of educational attainment on health outcomes through social experiences has also been the subject of much investigation. In the Egerter and colleagues model, educational attainment is posited to influence *social networks*, *social standing*, and *control beliefs*, each of which is assumed to affect health outcomes. Social networks, for example, provide access to resources and support that individuals may not have in isolation, and can promote healthful behaviors through social norms. Social standing may influence health outcomes through effects on perceived status as well as on network-level effects like access to relatively powerful or resource-granting people. Control beliefs—the degree of control that individuals perceive themselves to have over their own life circumstances—are also posited to affect health outcomes, particularly as influences on personal attributes (eg, confidence, perseverance, self-efficacy) and self-promoting versus self-harming behaviors.[5] Empirical evidence supports many of these links between education and social experiences as well as the existence of links between social experiences and health outcomes (see the article devoted to Margaret Fordham and colleagues' article, "the social context," later in this issue).

EDUCATION AS CONTEXT

In addition to educational attainment itself, schools provide an important context in which students spend a substantial portion of their time. The average U.S. school year is 180 days, and the minimum number of required hours for each of those days ranges from 3 to 6 hours depending on the state.[17] For students who enter a formal school system in kindergarten and exit after high school graduation, it is conceivable that those students have spent more than 14,000 hours in a school-based setting. Despite regulated school days and educational content, student experiences within these settings are highly variable, suggesting the presence of school-level determinants of outcomes.

Huang and colleagues suggest six domains in which school determinants of health can be organized.

- Physical and structural environment (eg, physical safety, air quality, hazardous environments, and rural/urban location)
- Health policies (eg, policies for health education and school safety)
- Health programs (eg, nutrition, physical education, prevention/intervention, and health services)
- Health resources (eg, availability of nurses, school counselors, and links between school and community health resources)
- School climate (eg, violence/bullying, school norms, teacher-child relationships)
- School composition (eg, average pupils' socio-economic status [SES], student and staff gender and racial/ethnic composition, and school size)

Their synthesis of this literature suggests that school determinants explain 4% to 40% of variance on pupils' health behaviors (eg, smoking habits and alcohol use). Variables related to school climate (eg, relationships between teachers and pupils) explain 5% to 8% of variance on pupils' well-being, and school physical education and fitness programs explain about 10% of variance on child health.[18]

For the purposes of this article, we focus on three of the more mutable determinants - health programs, health resources, and school climate. We will briefly take up the other three – physical and structural environment, school composition, and health policies - later in the article when we discuss how sociopolitical contexts affect school inequalities. This separation, however, should not suggest that some domains have positive influence and others negative; rather all six domains have the *potential* to affect short- and long-term health and wellbeing for students. At the same time, inequities among and within schools, which are often driven by broader inequities in race, class, ability, and geographic location, influence all of these domains and have the potential to exacerbate and amplify existing inequalities.[3]

Health Programs

Because the vast majority of U.S. children aged 5 to 18 attend public or private schools, school-based health curricula can be a powerful approach to increasing health-related knowledge and encouraging health-promoting behaviors. Kann and colleagues document the many different types of health curricula, including nutrition and healthy eating; tobacco, alcohol, and drug risks; mental health and psychological well-being; suicide prevention; violence prevention; and sexual health.[19] For example, most adolescents receive formal sexuality education from teachers or school nurses while in middle school and/or high school.[20] Although recent studies suggest that adolescents are more likely to seek sexual health information from friends, relatives, and media-based sources, school-based education programs can ensure more equitable access to accurate information that supports lifelong sexual health literacy and behavior.[21] Interventions that increase knowledge alone are insufficient to affect health outcomes, however. Rather, multiple studies suggest that school-based health programs are most effective when they involve multiple, reinforcing components (eg, knowledge improvement, behavior change, increased access to health-promoting resources), are implemented with fidelity, and exist for enough time to have durable effects.[22] High-quality implementation, of course, requires resources that may or may not be available in schools and certainly are distributed unequally among them.[18]

Health Services

Most U.S. schools provide basic health services (eg, height/weight measurements and hearing/eye tests), and most have school nurses and school counselors embedded within schools. School-based health professionals are especially well-positioned to mitigate some of the barriers to good health experienced by children and their families. They are easily accessible to children within the school setting, and lower some of the barriers that exist in accessing health and mental health care through traditional healthcare providers. For example, seeing a school nurse or school mental health professional does not require the student's parents to pay for services, take time off work, travel, or make an appointment.[23]

Noting the importance of school nurses in promoting school-based health and filling the gap in access to health services, the National Academy of Pediatrics recommended in 2016 that each school should have at least one full-time registered nurse to address student health needs.[24] Data from the National Teacher and Principal Survey demonstrate that this recommendation is far from realized. During 2015 to 16 academic year, only 52% of public schools had a full-time nurse, with schools that have a higher percentage of students qualifying for free and reduced lunch even less likely to have a school nurse.[25]

The same survey demonstrates that 94% of schools have some type of mental health worker (school counselor, school psychologist, social worker) on staff, and that these rates do not differ based on the racial or socioeconomic composition of the student body.[26] In fact, the survey revealed that schools in which the majority of students were part of a minoritized racial or ethnic group were slightly more likely to have a mental health professional on staff.[26] Despite this, 61% of schools claimed they had an insufficient number of mental health professionals necessary to manage the school's caseload, an issue especially impacting low-income schools.[26] Across the board, the caseloads of school mental health professionals significantly exceed recommendations by the American School Counseling Association (ASCA).[26] School nurses and mental health professionals are more likely to compensate for the absence of care from a PCP or non-school mental health professional rather than the other way around, however, a number of school-based health providers note the importance of partnerships among school-based and community-based health care providers for creating a more robust system of care.[27] Primary care providers, therefore, might seek to identify, participate in, and/or initiate partnerships in their communities; they might also advocate for the importance of school-based health care as a complementary service to community-based primary care.

School Climate

School climate is a multidimensional construct that includes real and perceived physical and emotional safety; the existence of engaged and supportive relationships; clearly defined norms and expectations for students; and student-teacher interactions within the instructional context.[28] Positive school climate is associated with a host of positive mental health outcomes, including lower anxiety, fewer depressive symptoms, and reductions in violent behavior and suicidal ideation.[29] Moreover, these outcomes persist across time[30] and demographic categories.[31] Like other markers of school quality, however, school climate is not equally distributed. For example, Voigt and colleagues' study of climate in schools across the state of California found that just as there is a racial attainment gap in education, there is also a "racial school environment gap."[32] Specifically, White and Asian students reported higher levels of safety, support, and connectedness at school when compared with Black, Native American, and Latino students. These differences were evident both between *and within* schools, meaning that even in schools with positive climates, students of color were less likely to feel safe or connected. Although the study authors were not focused on health outcomes, they do claim a causative role for school climate in school attainment, stating, "reducing racial disparities in students' experience of school climate will result in reduced racial disparities in achievement." One might reasonably surmise, therefore, that reducing racial disparities in students' experience of school climate might also play a role in reducing racial disparities in health.

Educators and education policy makers initially became interested in school climate because a positive school climate was shown to influence educational outcomes. Along the way, educators recognized the link between school climate and health, and the link between positive health and improved educational outcomes. Because of the reciprocal and reinforcing relationship between education and health, Dudovitz and colleagues argue that health providers and policy makers should take access to high-quality education and educational contexts seriously, just as educators and education policy makers should recognize the importance of health in contributing to educational success.[33] School climate can be challenging to change, but is possible, as researchers have demonstrated across various resource settings.[34]

EDUCATION AS DISTRIBUTED GOOD

The backdrop to all conversations about educational attainment and educational context and their influence on health is the reality that there are great disparities in accessing and using high-quality education just as there are disparities in health. We therefore propose the idea of conceptualizing education and educational contexts as distributed goods: goods that are currently distributed according to race, class, and ability status – among others – but could be distributed differently given the political will to do so. In claiming that education is a "distributed good," we echo the work of economist Amartya Sen and others who understand inequality not as an issue of scarcity, but rather as an issue of distribution.[35] In the U.S. context, the distribution of resources to education and educational contexts is driven by federal, state, and local policies, as well as existing social conditions such as persistent residential segregation based on race, class, and geography.[16] These lead to differences in school physical and social environments, school composition, and the ability of schools to implement and respond to broader health and educational policies. Zajacova and colleagues note that just as education and educational contexts can positively affect health and other opportunities, they can also reproduce inequality, and that interventions – scholarly and otherwise – into education as a social determinant of health must consider the sociopolitical contexts for which the education–health association is embedded.[3]

THE ROLE OF THE PRIMARY CARE PROVIDER IN SCREENING AND ADDRESSING EDUCATIONAL DETERMINANTS

Although addressing many of the above educational determinants is beyond the scope of the primary care provider (PCP), as discussed in other articles in this issue, the PCP still plays an important role in the lives of affected individuals. Screening for educational determinants and intervening when appropriate is an important part of addressing inequities. Screening can be done in routine annual pediatric exams and incorporated into standard HEADDSS screening (*H*ome, *E*ducation/Employment, Peer Group *A*ctivities, *D*iet/Drugs, *S*exuality, and *S*uicide/depression). If suboptimal determinants are uncovered, patient and caregiver education can then be done to heighten awareness, enabling more informed caretaker participation in corrective activities. PCP intervention might also be appropriate in certain cases, when for example, educational determinants associated with depression or behavioral issues are uncovered. In sum, it is important for the PCP to screen for educational determinants, educate and intervene as needed, and refer to outside agencies when appropriate.

CLINICS CARE POINTS

- Interventions that improve patients' health literacy and ability to access and evaluate accurate health information are a necessary step in improving patient outcomes. Clinicians should consider *directing patients to reputable sources of on-line health information and recommending best practices when evaluating health information*, along with providing standard patient education materials and encouragement to contact health care providers with concerns and questions.

- When child or adolescent patients present with symptoms of depression and anxiety, *clinicians should be open to discussing the school context* as a possible source and/or contributor to these symptoms, as well as a possible resource upon which to draw support and services.
- *Developing child and adolescent treatment plans in collaboration with caregivers, educators, and social service providers* is best practice when treating children with complex and/or persistent health needs.
- Clinicians should be *mindful of school environment in addition to home environment when understanding a child's health risks.* For example, school air quality could be exacerbating asthma symptoms; the availability of physical education and sports team opportunities could help or hinder physical activity levels; and the presence of school nurses and counselors – while an asset when available – should not be assumed.

COI AND FUNDING DISCLOSURE

Authors do not have any commercial or financial conflicts of interest to disclose. Both authors and the work on this article are funded in part by National Cancer Institute, United States U54 CA163072.

REFERENCES

1. Case A, Deaton A. Life expectancy in adulthood is falling for those without a BA degree, but as educational gaps have widened, racial gaps have narrowed. Proc Natl Acad Sci U S A 2021;118(11). e2024777118.
2. Hess A., (March 19, 2021). College graduates live longer than those without a college degree—and the gap is growing. Available at: https://www.cnbc.com/2021/03/19/college-graduates-live-longer-than-those-without-a-college-degree.html. Accessed January 23, 2023.
3. Zajacova A, Lawrence EM. The Relationship Between Education and Health: Reducing Disparities Through a Contextual Approach. Annu Rev Public Health 2018;39(1):273–89.
4. McCarthy ML, Zheng Z, Wilder ME, et al. Latent Class Analysis to Represent Social Determinant of Health Risk Groups in the Medicaid Cohort of the District of Columbia. Med Care 2021;59(3):251–8.
5. Egerter S, Braveman P, Sadegh-Nobari T, et al. Education matters for health. Exploring the social determinants of health (Issue brief no. 5). Princeton, NJ: Robert Wood Johnson Foundation; 2011.
6. Teles M, Kaya S. Health literacy of cardiology patients: determinants and effects on patient outcomes. Soc Work Health Care 2021;60(10):656–73.
7. Damiani G, Basso D, Acampora A, et al. The impact of level of education on adherence to breast and cervical cancer screening: Evidence from a systematic review and meta-analysis. Prev Med 2015;81:281–9.
8. Fletcher JM, Frisvold DE. Higher Education and Health Investments: Does More Schooling Affect Preventive Health Care Use? J Hum Cap 2009;3(2):144–76.
9. Berkman ND, Sheridan SL, Donahue KE, et al. Low Health Literacy and Health Outcomes: An Updated Systematic Review. Ann Intern Med 2011;155(2):97–107.
10. Margolis R. Educational Differences in Healthy Behavior Changes and Adherence Among Middle-aged Americans. J Health Soc Behav 2013;54(3):353–68.
11. Jackson MI, Kihara T. The Educational Gradient in Health Among Children in Immigrant Families. Popul Res Pol Rev 2019;38:869–97.

12. Artiga S, Hinton E. Beyond health care: the role of social determinants in promoting health and health equity (Issue brief). San Francisco, CA: Henry J. Kaiser Family Foundation; 2018.
13. Case A, Fertig A, Paxson C. The Lasting Impact of Childhood Health and Circumstance. J Health Econ 2005;24(2):365–89.
14. Clougherty JE, Souza K, Cullen MR. Work and its role in shaping the social gradient in health. Ann N Y Acad Sci 2010;1186(1):102–24.
15. Parker Ms, Bucknall M, Jagger C, et al. Population-based estimates of healthy working life expectancy in England at age 50 years: analysis of data from the English Longitudinal Study of Ageing. Lancet Public Health 2020;5:e395–403.
16. Johnson R. The Health Returns of Education Policies from Preschool to High School and Beyond. Am Econ Rev 2010;100:188–94.
17. National Center for Education Statistics, U.S. Department of Education (2020). State Education Practices. Available at: https://nces.ed.gov/programs/statereform/tab1_1-2020.asp. Accessed January 23, 2023.
18. Huang KY, Cheng S, Theise R. School Contexts as Social Determinants of Child Health: Current Practices and Implications for Future Public Health Practice. Publ Health Rep 2013;128(Suppl 3):21–8.
19. Kann L, Telljohann SK, Wooley SF. Health Education: Results from the School Health Policies and Programs Study 2006. J Sch Health 2007;77(8):408–34.
20. National Center for Health Statistics (2010). NCHS Data Brief: Educating Teenagers about Sex in the United States. Available at: www.cdc.gov/nchs/data/databriefs/db44.htm. Accessed January 23, 2023.
21. Graf A, Hicks Patrick J. Foundations of life-long sexual health literacy. Health Education; 2015. p. 115. https://doi.org/10.1108/HE-12-2013-0073.
22. Foster GD, Sherman S, Borradaile KE, et al. A Policy-Based School Intervention to Prevent Overweight and Obesity. Pediatrics 2008;121(4):e794–802.
23. Schroeder K, Malone S, McCabe E, et al. Addressing the Social Determinants of Health: A Call to Action for School Nurses. J Sch Nurs 2018;34. 105984051775073.
24. Council on School Health, Holmes BW, Sheetz A, et al. Role of the School Nurse in Providing School Health Services. Pediatrics 2016;137(6). e20160852.
25. National Center for Education Statistics, U.S. Department of Education (2020). Data Point: School Nurses in Public Schools. Available at: https://nces.ed.gov/pubs2020/2020086/index.asp. Accessed January 23, 2023.
26. National Center for Education Statistics, U.S. Department of Education (2019). Data Point: Mental Health Staff in Public Schools, by School Racial and Ethnic Composition. Available at: https://nces.ed.gov/pubs2019/2019020/index.asp. Accessed January 23, 2023.
27. Atkins M, Cappella E, Shernoff T, et al. Schooling and Children's Mental Health: Realigning Resources to Reduce Disparities and Advance Public Health. Annu Rev Clin Psychol 2017;13:123–47.
28. National School Climate Center. (no date). School Climate. Available at: https://schoolclimate.org/school-climate/. Accessed January 23, 2023.
29. Center for Social and Emotional Education. School climate research summary—January 2010. Available at: http://www.schoolclimate.org/climate/documents/SCBrief_v1n1_Jan2010.pdf. Accessed January 23, 2023.
30. Wong MD, Dosanjh KK, Jackson NJ, et al. The Longitudinal Relationship of School Climate with Adolescent Social and Emotional Health. BMC Publ Health 2021;21:207.

31. Franco K, Baumler E, Torres ED, et al. The link between school climate and mental health among an ethnically diverse sample of middle school youth. Curr Psychol 2022.
32. Voight A. The Racial School-Climate Gap. San Francisco: WestEd; 2013. A report from the region IX equity Assistance Center at WestEd.
33. Dudovitz RN, Nelson BB, Coker TR, et al. Long-term Health Implications of School Quality. Soc Sci Med 2016;158:1–7.
34. Bradshaw CP, Koth CW, Thornton LA, et al. Altering School Climate through School-Wide Positive Behavioral Interventions and Supports: Findings from a Group-Randomized Effectiveness Trial. Prev Sci 2009;10:100–15.
35. Sen A. Development as freedom. New York, NY: Oxford University Press; 1999.

The Built Environment as a Social Determinant of Health

Rosemary Nabaweesi, MBChB, DrPH[a,*], Marie Hanna, MD[b], John K. Muthuka, PhD[c], Adrian D. Samuels, PhD[a], Vanisha Brown, PhD, MPH[d], Dawn Schwartz, MEd[e], Green Ekadi, PhD[d]

KEYWORDS

• Built environment • Racism • Health disparities • Housing quality

KEY POINTS

- The built environment contributes significantly to one's health and well-being both mentally and physically.
- The built environment our patients reside in, work in, and play and learn in largely depends on their race and socioeconomic status.
- When managing patients, consider the patient's-built environment at home, workplace, school, and respective neighborhood and mechanisms affecting their health: indoor microbiome, neighborhood effects, toxins, injury risks, safety or security, and walkability.

INTRODUCTION

The built environment touches all aspects of our lives. It encompasses the buildings we live in; the distribution systems that provide us with water and electricity; and the roads, bridges, and transportation systems we use to get from place to place. Significant health disparities across disease manifestations and associated structural racism in our society highlight the need for an in-depth examination of the built environment as a social determinant of health (SDOH). This article will discuss the

[a] Center for Health Policy, School of Graduate Studies, Meharry Medical College, 1005 Dr. D. B. Todd Jr. Boulevard, Nashville, TN 37208, USA; [b] Family Medicine, PGY-3, Meharry Medical College, 1005 Dr. D. B. Todd Jr. Boulevard, Nashville, TN 37208, USA; [c] Kenya Medical Training College, PO Box 30195-00100, Nairobi, Kenya; [d] School of Graduate Studies, Meharry Medical College, 1005 Dr. D. B. Todd Jr. Boulevard, Nashville, TN 37208, USA; [e] Department of Health Policy, Vanderbilt University Medical Center, 2525 West End Avenue, Suite 1201, Nashville, TN 37203, USA
* Corresponding author.
E-mail address: rnabaweesi@mmc.edu
Twitter: @rnabawe1 (R.N.); @johnmuthuka1 (J.K.M.)

Prim Care Clin Office Pract 50 (2023) 591–599
https://doi.org/10.1016/j.pop.2023.04.012
primarycare.theclinics.com

historical and social-political events that shaped the nation's built infrastructure at its inception and how local, state, and federal policies have consolidated neighborhood segregation.

The article describes the impact one's physical environment has on their well-being, both physically and mentally, through direct or indirect mechanisms. We discuss public health effects including safety, health, physical and psychological trauma, and adverse childhood experiences (ACEs). It is important that physicians understand the historical and sociopolitical contexts that frame the built environments in the catchment areas they serve. The article will explore opportunities and options that primary care physicians can use to help improve patient outcomes within their built environment to improve overall health status, minimize health risks, and speed recovery from ill health.

The Built Environment

The built environment can be described as the man-made or modified structures that provide people with living, working, and recreational spaces.[1] The built environment is meant to provide safety, health, wellbeing and meaning to its dwellers, as a place to rest, work, live, learn, play, and thrive.[2,3] In the twentieth century, the American Public Health Association developed a report on the *Basic Principles of Healthy Housing*[4] identifying 30 principles to cover people's physiological and psychological health and protect them from infections and injuries. Several recommended measurements and requirements are still applicable in today's housing design and embedded in the building codes. The 5 primary performance indicators for healthy buildings today originated from APHA's Basic Principles of Healthy Housing: (1) thermal environment, (2) indoor air environment, (3) daylight and lighting environment, (4) noise, and (5) safety. Lately, healthy building performance indicators are more focused on physiological indicators, due to an increased understanding of factors affecting overall human performance and cover lighting, thermal comfort, personal security, ventilation, and moisture control. As housing is generally regarded as a cardinal SDOH.[5] physicians should endeavor to understand, investigate and work to mitigate these issues that relate to the overall health of their patients.

Negative physical health effects of poor housing include toxins within the home, mold, cold indoor temperatures, and overcrowding among other safety factors, all of which need to be explored more during the limited time physicians have with their patients. The negative mental health effects of a poor built environment have been documented even more extensively because it has been linked to stress, depression, and anxiety.[6]

The adverse impacts of health disparities and structural elements of racism over the life span of our society highlight the need for an in-depth examination of the built environment as a SDOH. Although further research is needed on the effects of a built environment on a patient, given the evidence that does exist, it is adamant that primary care physicians incorporate exploring environmental impacts on their patients' health into the clinical care visit.

History: the Creation of Racially Segregated Residential Neighborhoods

White and minoritized families have generally lived segregated lives throughout American history. Black and White families were segregated throughout history because of racist ideologies and policies. Three types of federal, state policies and practices were designed to introduce racial segregation in previously integrated neighborhoods while reinforcing racial segregation in others.[7,8] These policies further linked racial and economic segregation by concentrating Black poverty and White affluence across the country. The policies include (1) public housing, (2) exclusionary and industrial zoning, and (3) redlining.[8,9]

The first public housing developments for civilians were created as part of the New Deal under President Roosevelt to address housing shortages from the Great Depression and World War II. These were meant for lower middle-class White families and were not subsidized. After World War II, the G.I. Bill was passed to assist returning veterans and better position them to take advantage of the booming postwar economy. One main provision of the G.I. Bill was low interest loans to veterans to increase home ownership. However, Black war veterans were denied the wholesale benefits of the G.I. Bill. Instead, Black families seeking mortgages faced discriminatory practices from local lenders and home insurers that prevented access to home loans or forced them to accept loans at much higher interest rates than comparable White families. For those who did qualify, they were denied purchasing homes in White neighborhoods with racial covenants and redlining, which is denying a home loan or insurance to someone who lives in an economically undesirable area.

With the inability to gain home ownership, many Black families moved to White vacated public housing developments, which also accelerated "white flight" to the suburbs. The 1949 Housing Act enacted under President Truman increased public housing across the country including the development of massive, high-rise residential buildings in many cities. Although public housing became available to more Black families, the Housing Act promoted and consolidated racial segregation of the units with increased capacity and access, as greater divides between White and Black neighborhoods were strengthened with legislative, business, and social policies.[10,11]

As the housing market across America became more racially divided in the mid-twentieth century, the real estate industry lobbied to severely limit the reach of public housing. Subsequent new regulation imposed strict upper-income limits to qualify for public housing, transforming it into concentrated areas of inner-city poverty.[10,12] With the growing supply of housing in the 1950s, there was a cultural shift toward suburban, single-family home ownership, supported by other favorable government actions, such as the construction of the interstate system, which added to "white flight" from metropolitan areas.

This cultural and structural shift not only relegated public housing to the poor but also relegated specifically to poor Black families. The loss of middle-class rents to support public housing also brought about severe reductions in maintenance budgets.[12] The latter explains the building dilapidation associated with public housing, confining minority mostly Black families to poorly maintained housing. Racial residential segregation not only meant separate in physical location but also systematically unequal.[13] Segregation based on racial differences has been linked to numerous causes of racial disparity and inequalities, with educational attainment and economic mobility being the chief contributors.[14]

SHAPED BY LAW AND GOVERNMENTAL DECISIONS

Built environment for residential and commercial use is governed by a complex set of local, state, and federal laws. Current inner-city residential neighborhoods are based on outdated racist urban land use practices codified into law in 1933 with the Home Owner's Loan Act. The act established the Federal Home Owner Lending Corporation designations for assigning parcel values and more specifically the bias of lending only to White suburban families.[15,16] Residential segregation was legitimized and adjudicated through structures of government, finance, home sales, and zoning, a practice known as "redlining."[17] Although this legal practice was struck down in the 1960s, existing health inequities/disparities map directly onto the historical redlined regions.

It is costly to ensure all housing standards are met. People experiencing poverty, such as communities with historical deinvestment are left with few options but to live in substandard housing, couch surf or remain unhoused. Substandard housing affects inhabitants' physical and mental health, and well-being via various mechanisms including indoor microbiome, chemical, neighborhood effects, and physical and social factors.[6,18]

Evidence shows that cost-burdened households are prevalent among low-income and minority populations.[19] Cost-burdened is defined as spending more than 30% of Average Median household Income on housing costs. Cost-burdened shares are much higher among Black (45%) and Hispanic households (43%) than among Asian and other minority households (36%) or White households (27%). Additionally, within the same income group, larger shares of minority groups are cost burdened.

Connection of Housing to Physical and Mental Health

Built environment affects health-related outcomes through various domains including land use, street environment, transportation infrastructure, green and open spaces, and neighborhood facilities.[20] The main built environmental factors that determine peoples' health development, health challenges, and health equity include accessibility and quality of housing. Evidence shows that substandard housing features, which are common in public housing, for example, lack of hot water, safe drinking water, effective waste disposals, and pest infestation contribute to spread of infection.[3,21] Studies have shown that significant health disparities documented in asthma and other chronic respiratory diseases are associated with damp, cold, moldy housing even after controlling for income, smoking, and overcrowding.[6,19,22] Water intrusion from interior and exterior leaks is the major cause of dampness. Overcrowding and poor ventilation are the other contributors. The mechanism of respiratory illness is through mites, roaches, molds, and viruses, all of which thrive on damp environments. Pest infestation particularly roaches and mites have been shown to cause allergenic sensitization and thus asthmatic triggers.[23]

A second attribute of hazardous housing is chemicals such as lead, asbestos, radon, carbon monoxide, and tobacco smoke carcinogens.[24,25] Literature presents strong evidence associating poor mental health to disadvantaged neighborhood's built environments with examples such as unclean air (radon) and water (Flint lead crisis) unsafe, insecure neighborhoods, which also threaten children's and their families' physical health, and safety.[6,26–28] There is evidence to show that residents living in disadvantaged neighborhoods have higher rates of stress, cancer, and depression.[29,30]

Adverse Childhood Experiences

According to the Centers for Disease Control and Prevention, ACEs are potentially traumatic events that occur during childhood and include witnessing violence, having a parent imprisoned or dying, substance abuse, and racism. ACEs have been shown to occur at higher rates among people living in conditions of poverty, in neighborhoods with high crime rates, and high levels of exclusion from economic investment.[31]

Evidence shows that experiencing more than 3 ACEs predisposes people to chronic metabolic diseases such as addictions, obesity, cardiovascular disease, and other behavioral challenges such as difficulty with learning resulting in poor educational outcomes. Promoting safe, stable nurturing environments and relationships where children live, grow, learn, and play reduces the likelihood of multiple ACEs occurring.

Effectively healing influenced communities entails restoring and maintaining the roads, parks, buildings, and transportation infrastructure so that they can foster positive social interaction with economic mobility and safety.[3,11,25,32]

Psychological trauma: impact of chronic and toxic stress on health

Types of building (eg, high rise), floor level and overall housing quality have been associated with mental health changes in dwellers such as depression, anxiety, negative affect, and behavioral disturbances. Mothers with young children (**Fig. 1**) living in high-rise multiple unit dwellings report various degrees of psychological distress. Possible explanations for this association are the social isolation and limited play opportunities for children as well as safety concerns for their children (eg, predisposition to falls).[28] Women in large high-rise buildings (old style project housing) report higher levels of loneliness and diminished territorial control than their counterparts residing in different housing types.

There is an inverse association between housing quality and psychological distress.[6,23] Sound housing structural quality, maintenance and upkeep, amenities are associated with mental well-being (**Fig. 2**). Although studies on mental health and built environment are mostly cross-sectional, and rely on self-reports, research shows that when people move to better housing their mental health improves.[3,33,34] Some of the explanations for the housing quality affecting mental health include insecurity associated with low-quality housing, unresponsive landlords, and unending disrepair.[6,18,23] Lack of affordable housing means people with low-incomes relocate frequently and are forced to live in undesirable environments. Involuntary relocation not only causes stress in adults but also affects psychological adjustment.[18,28,35] Frequent relocations have been reported to cause socioemotional problems among children.[6,28]

DISCUSSION

Neighborhoods with concentrated poverty are defined as areas where 30% or more of the residents live in households whose income is below the Federal poverty line.

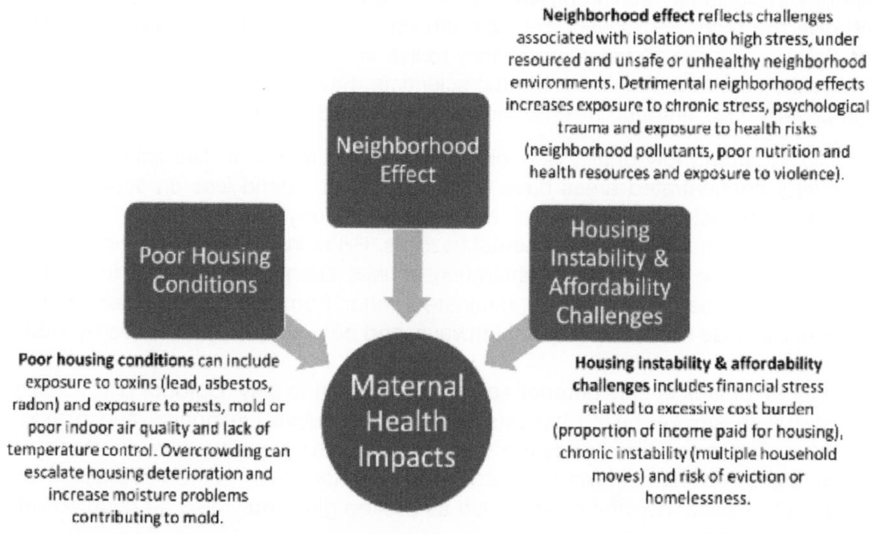

Fig. 1. Housing pathways that affect infant and maternal health. (*From* Reece J. More Than Shelter: Housing for Urban Maternal and Infant Health. Int J Environ Res Public -37782550863500Health. 2021;18(7):3331. Published 2021 Mar 24.)

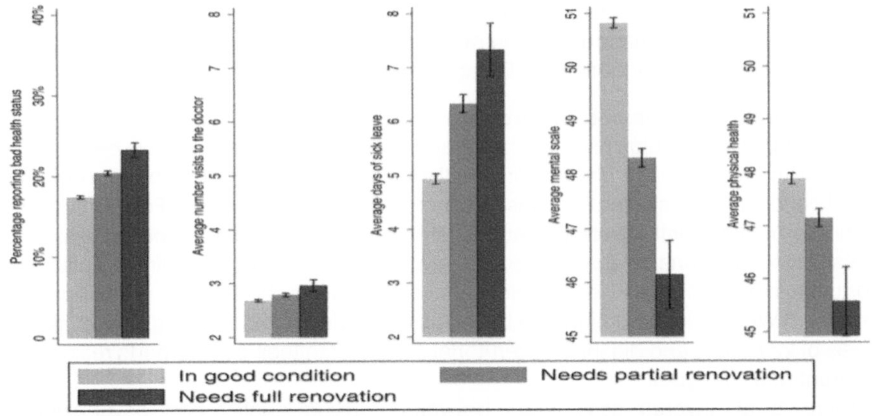

Fig. 2. Housing conditions and occupant health. (*From* Palacios, J, Eichholtz, P, Kok, N, Aydin, E. The impact of housing conditions on health outcomes. Real Estate Econ. 2021; 49: 1172–1200.)

Neighborhoods with concentrated poverty are a common occurrence across the country and are found in both large and small metropolitan cities. Overall, about 6.7% of the US population lives in these neighborhoods, whereas 12.5% of Hispanic population and 20% of African Americans live in such neighborhoods. The Pew Charitable Trust has shown a link between high-concentrated poverty neighborhoods and downward mobility, higher rates of mobility (unstable housing), unemployment, poor-quality schools, and increased violence and resulting threats to families' economic security.[15,22,36]

Segregated housing came into being initially by historical local, state, and federal housing policies that intentionally discriminated against Black and Brown people and discouraged investment in particular communities. These policies along with present day exclusionary zoning policies create neighborhoods of concentrated poverty and disadvantage. Segregation by race, ethnicity, and income are often intertwined, and Black youth are 10 times more likely to live in disadvantaged communities than their White counterparts. Child Trends' scientists, have shown that children living in high poverty-concentrated neighborhoods are harmed via these 5 mechanisms.

1. Children attend low-quality schools beginning in preschool. The schools in high poverty-concentrated areas have fewer resources, spend less on staffing, have inadequate instructional material, and have worse physical buildings.
2. High concentration of environmental hazards. Risks inside the home include hazards associate with older, deteriorating houses such as mold, pest infestation, and peeling lead paint and contaminated water from lead pipes. Risks outside the home arise from proximity to highways, and poor air quality from nearby industrial sources.
3. Reduced or lack of safe outdoor spaces for children to play. Outdoor play is associated with several health benefits including executive functioning and physical fitness. These neighborhoods are more likely to have unsafe parks, sports fields, biking and walking trails, and playgrounds if they have them in the first place. Presence of physical harmful effects such as broken glass may also be coupled with environmental hazards.
4. Children are more likely to experience ACEs such as violence, imprisonment of a parent, neglect (physical or emotional). These traumatic events can trigger

powerful stress responses in children resulting in lifetime impacts such as obesity, depression, and addictions.
5. Significantly reduced likelihood of economic mobility.

SUMMARY

The built environment contributes significantly to one's health and well-being both mentally and physically. The built environment our patients reside in, work in, and play and learn in largely depends on their race and socioeconomic status. When managing patients, consider the patient's built environment at home, workplace, school, and respective neighborhood and mechanisms affecting their health: indoor microbiome, neighborhood effects, toxins, injury risks, safety or security, and walkability.

CLINICS CARE POINTS

Consider the following risks when evaluating your patients' clinical condition and provide anticipatory guidance accordingly.

- Physical injury inside or outside the home, workplace, or school
- Exposure to toxins inside the built environment (home/work/school)
- Environmental hazards such as motor vehicle crashes, pedestrian struck, chemical exposures, air pollution, and broken glass in playgrounds
- ACEs
- Recommend social work services when patient is experiencing housing challenges
- Collaborate with your public health departments and divisions to tap into resources such as Health Homes programs by home visitors

Advocate for your patients in these areas.

1. Deimplement harmful policies
2. Implement equitable policies
3. Correct historical injustice

Health-care organizations are encouraged to support community investments that improve built environment conditions and promote physical and mental health for all populations across the life span.

DISCLOSURE

The authors have nothing to disclose.

REFERENCES

1. Basic Information about Built Environment. Available at; https://www.epa.gov/smm/basic-information-about-built-environment. Accessed February 28, 2022.
2. Hu M, Roberts JD. Connections and Divergence between Public Health and Built Environment—A Scoping Review. Urban Science 2020;4(1):12.
3. Krieger J, Higgins DL, Housing, et al. Time Again for Public Health Action. Am J Public Health 2002;92(5):758–68.
4. Winslow CEA, Adams FJ, Britten RH, et al. Basic Principles of Healthful Housing. Am J Public Health Nation's Health 1938;28(3):351–72.

5. Rolfe S, Garnham L, Godwin J, et al. Housing as a social determinant of health and wellbeing: developing an empirically-informed realist theoretical framework. BMC Publ Health 2020;20(1):1138.
6. Holding E, Blank L, Crowder M, et al. Exploring the relationship between housing concerns, mental health and wellbeing: a qualitative study of social housing tenants. J Public Health 2020;42(3):e231–8.
7. Hanley J. The color of law: A forgotten history of how our government segregated America. J Urban Aff 2019;41(8):0. https://doi.org/10.1080/07352166.2019.1588576.
8. Shapiro A, Rothstein R. The Color Of Law' Details How U.S. Housing Policies Created Segregation. Published online May 17, 2017.
9. Chapin T. Rothstein: The Color of Law: A Forgotten History of How Our Government Segregated America. J Am Plann Assoc 2020;86(4):516–7.
10. 1933: The New Deal and the Home Owner's Loan Corporation (HOLC). Accessed March 30, 2023. 1933: The New Deal and the Home Owner's Loan Corporation (HOLC).
11. Miller WD, Pollack CE, Williams DR. Healthy Homes and CommunitiesPutting the Pieces Together. Am J Prev Med 2011;40(1):S48–57.
12. Housing Discrimination Against Racial And Ethnic Minorities 2012. Available at: https://www.huduser.gov/portal/publications/fairhsg/hsg_discrimination_2012.html. Accessed March 30, 2023.
13. Browman AS, Destin M, Kearney MS, et al. How economic inequality shapes mobility expectations and behaviour in disadvantaged youth. Nat Hum Behav 2019;3(3):214–20.
14. Williams DR. Racial residential segregation: a fundamental cause of racial disparities in health. Publ Health Rep 2001;116(5):404–16.
15. Chaskin RJ. Integration and Exclusion. Ann Am Acad Pol Soc Sci 2013;647(1):237–67.
16. Swope CB, Hernández D, Cushing LJ. The relationship of historical redlining with present-day neighborhood environmental and health outcomes: a scoping review and conceptual model. J Urban Health 2022;99(6):959–83.
17. Gale DE. Review: *The Color of Law: A Forgotten History of How Our Government Segregated America* by Richard Rothstein. J Plan Educ Res 2019;39(3):380–1.
18. Goetz EG. Desegregation in 3D: Displacement, Dispersal and Development in American Public Housing. Hous Stud 2010;25(2):137–58.
19. Apgar W, Brown H. The state of the nation's housing 1988-2018. Joint Center for Housing Studies of Harvard University; 1988.
20. Frank LD, Sallis JF, Conway TL, et al. Many Pathways from Land Use to Health: Associations between Neighborhood Walkability and Active Transportation, Body Mass Index, and Air Quality. J Am Plann Assoc 2006;72(1):75–87.
21. Martinez-Torteya C, Donovan A, Gilchrist MA, et al. Neighborhood disadvantage moderates the effect of perinatal intimate partner violence (IPV) exposure on disorganized attachment behaviors among 12-month-old infants. Psychol Violence 2021;11(1):101–11.
22. Bashir SA. Home Is Where the Harm Is: Inadequate Housing as a Public Health Crisis. Am J Public Health 2002;92(5):733–8.
23. Marsh A, Gordon D, Heslop P, et al. Housing Deprivation and Health: A Longitudinal Analysis. Hous Stud 2000;15(3):411–28.
24. Taylor D. Environmental Racism, Industrial Pollution, and Residential Mobility. Nat Resour J 2014;55(1):701–4.

25. Hilovsky K, Kenneth L, Williams T. Creating The Healthiest Nation: Health and Housing Equity; 2020.
26. Gandolff R. Lead exposure in childhood and historical land use: a geostatistical analysis of soil lead concentrations in South Philadelphia parks. Environ Monit Assess 2023;195(3):356.
27. Lodge EK, Guseh NS, Martin CL, et al. The effect of residential proximity to brownfields, highways, and heavy traffic on serum metal levels in the Detroit Neighborhood Health Study. Environmental Advances 2022;9:100278.
28. Evans GW. The Built Environment and Mental Health. J Urban Health 2003;80(4): 536–55.
29. Nilsen FM, Ruiz JDC, Tulve NS. A Meta-Analysis of Stressors from the Total Environment Associated with Children's General Cognitive Ability. Int J Environ Res Public Health 2020;17(15):5451.
30. Saleem FT, Busby DR, Lambert SF. Neighborhood social processes as moderators between racial discrimination and depressive symptoms for African American adolescents. J Community Psychol 2018;46(6):747–61.
31. Center for Disease Control and Prevention: Adverse Childhood Experiences. Published April 2021. Available at: www.Cdc.Gov/Violenceprevention/Aces/Index.Html. Accessed March 30, 2023.
32. Mantler T, Jackson KT, Walsh EJ, et al. Promoting Attachment Through Healing (PATH): Results of a retrospective feasibility study providing trauma-and-violence-informed care to pregnant women. J Adv Nurs 2022;78(2):557–68.
33. de Souza Briggs X. Moving up versus moving out: Neighborhood effects in housing mobility programs. Hous Policy Debate 1997;8(1):195–234.
34. Sullivan AL, Lietz CA. Benefits and Risks for Public Housing Adolescents Experiencing Hope VI Revitalization: A Qualitative Study. J Poverty 2008;12(2):133–54.
35. Kearns A, Mason P. Defining and Measuring Displacement: Is Relocation from Restructured Neighbourhoods Always Unwelcome and Disruptive? Hous Stud 2013;28(2):177–204.
36. Ewing R, Cervero R. Travel and the Built Environment. J Am Plann Assoc 2010; 76(3):265–94.

The Social Context: Social and Behavioral Factors That Affect Health Outcomes

Jacqueline M. Hirth, PhD, MPH*, Sandra J. Gonzalez, PhD, MSSW, Roger Zoorob, MD, MPH

KEYWORDS

- Social support • Social networks • Stigma • Allostatic load • Social isolation

KEY POINTS

- Social support works through multiple mechanisms to affect mental and physical health outcomes.
- Family care practitioners may provide resources to increase support for patients with mental and physical health conditions to contribute to improved health outcomes.
- Approaches to reducing stigma in health care are available to contribute to improved patient care.
- The family care practitioner is a component of their patient's social network who can contribute to improving health through recommendations for tangible resources as well as related to increasing social contact and engagement.

MAKING THE CONNECTION: ALLOSTATIC LOAD AND HEALTH

The social environment affects mental and physical health through several possible routes, including stress. *Allostatic load* refers to the cumulative effect of exposure to stress over time that may promote biological dysregulation, which contributes to wear and tear through chronically overworked physiologic systems that are involved in the stress response.[1] This concept is commonly measured using biomarkers such as heart rate, blood pressure, glycosylated hemoglobin A1c, high-density lipoprotein (HDL) cholesterol, and C-reactive protein.[2] High levels of allostatic load are associated with a number of poor health conditions across the lifespan, including cancer, poor mental health, and periodontal disease.[3] Allostatic load may both cause poor health conditions and exacerbate existing conditions and has long been intertwined with the positive and negative benefits of social interactions within an individual's social environment. These interactions may have the result of either exacerbating

Department of Family and Community Medicine, Baylor College of Medicine, One Baylor Plaza, Houston, TX 77098, USA
* Corresponding author.
E-mail address: Jacqueline.hirth@bcm.edu

Prim Care Clin Office Pract 50 (2023) 601–620
https://doi.org/10.1016/j.pop.2023.04.008

existing stress or relieving it, thus contributing to or subtracting from the allostatic load burden an individual experiences.

The *social environment* includes several concepts and transactions—the exchange of information and both tangible and intangible support—that make up a person's experience of their connections between themselves and others. *Intangible support* is a type of support that may not be easily measured, such as spending time with or listening to another person. The social environment includes all physical surroundings, social relationships, and cultural settings which people function within.[4] Social structures within an individual's social environment are measured in several different ways, reflecting positive and negative interactions as well as the exchange of physical, monetary, emotional, and intangible support. Health care providers who understand the social environment within which their patients live can help to determine the care that is best for them and that patients will be able to maintain preventive or therapeutic medical regimens.

To achieve this understanding and best care, screening and treating patients should take into context the patient's social environment and how a patient receives support from others, including their health care team. Although contact may be limited between patients and their providers, the relationship that forms is important to care and management of disease and general screening. For example, older adults with type II diabetes may not be aware of the seriousness of their condition or even understand how nonadherence with treatment may affect their health due to poor communication between patient and provider.[5]

What are the Types of Social Connections and How are They Measured?

Measuring social relationships is a complex undertaking that requires careful consideration of the underlying construct. For example, the size and composition of an individual's social network has been associated with outcomes such as physical well-being, obesity, hypertension, and diabetes.[6,7] A study of adolescents found that friends tended to have a similar body mass index within their friend network, even after adjusting for home, school, and neighborhood factors.[8] Although these findings could be due to peer groups selecting for those with similar physical characteristics, they also indicate potential for stigma and other selection factors that may contribute to positive and negative social interactions that influence health across the life course. *Social support* is the emotional, instrumental (goods and services), and financial support obtained by an individual's social network and includes a transaction between 2 or more people.[9] *Social capital* is the collective resources that arise from social networks, usually within communities or in other group context.

Positive social relationships have long been known to be a benefit to the health of individuals across the lifespan.[1] *Social networks* are the "web of social ties that surrounds an individual."[9] Social networks are often measured by examining the structural dimensions of an individual's network. For example, it is important to consider the density and complexity, the size, the symmetry or reciprocity, geographic proximity, homogeneity, and accessibility of social network members.[9] Each of these components can be used to describe the types and frequency of social ties an individual has and which contributes to an individual's support from their network. Social network analysis does not concentrate on the characteristics of those within a network, but rather on the links between individuals.[9]

Social support affects health both directly and through stress buffering.[10] For example, individuals may adopt attitudes, beliefs, and behaviors based on comparisons of how others in their social network behave.[10] These norms affect health behaviors through observation of what is acceptable or appropriate within their group and can influence both positive and negative health behaviors. In a longitudinal study of over 12,000 people, the odds of developing obesity increased 57% if a friend became obese.[11] There were also increases in risk of developing obesity between siblings and spouses.[11] Increased social support is also associated with improved health behavior. A study of relapse in a study of participants with substance use disorders demonstrated that increased social support was associated with lower risk of relapse even if those providing social support used the same substance as the recovering subjects' problem substance.[12] As a result of strong associations between social support and relapse, a strong social support system is indicated as a consideration in the decision on who receives liver transplants for patients with alcoholic cirrhosis in many health care systems.[13]

Social support measures often include multiple components of social relationships even if they are fleeting or infrequent.[14] Social support may be measured differently depending on anticipated or actual needs for a population. For example, the social support needs of an older adult, who may need support for transportation or acquiring and retaining information among other needs, may be very different than an individual with obesity who is working to lose weight.[15,16] Thus, measures for social support tend to be individualized for different health conditions and life stages. Although different types of social support may be more supportive for different circumstances, it is often measured broadly using 2 concepts: tangible components such as financial support and physical aid as well as through intangible components including encouragement and guidance.[17]

Social engagement has long been considered a social determinant of health. Engagement with community activities, religious functions, employment, volunteering, and other activities that enable social connections to form have many ties to improved cardiovascular health, for example, particularly among middle-aged and older adults.[18–21] Cognitive decline and risk of Alzheimer's disease and other dementias are negatively associated with improved social engagement.[22]

Religious engagement or attendance at church-related activities and even spirituality is one area of social engagement that has been extensively studied as a social determinant of health.[23] These concepts are multi-dimensional, and may include both public and private practices, social support from an individual's religious community, commitment, forgiveness, daily spiritual experience, coping, beliefs and values, and overall self-ranking of level of religiosity or spiritual belief.[23] Numerous studies have linked this type of social engagement to better health outcomes and improved survival.[23] It is believed that improved health among those with greater levels of religious engagement or spirituality may work through improved optimism or even lifestyle modification related to social norms (eg, low substance use disorder rates and smoking among those with higher levels of religious engagement), and sharing of resources through extensive social networks.[23] Although religiosity has been extensively studied apart from social engagement, it likely works through similar mechanisms.

EFFECTS OF SOCIAL ENVIRONMENT ON ALLOSTATIC LOAD

The lifetime accumulation of allostatic load has repercussions on mental and physical health that contribute to increased mortality at younger ages.[24] Impaired mental health may also inhibit adaptation to stressors. Depression and anxiety symptoms among individuals who have not been diagnosed for those conditions may experience either exaggerated cortisol responses to stress or increased time for recovery after experiencing a stressor compared with those without the same symptoms.[25] A positive social environment, such as supportive and intimate relationships, has been established as having protective effects on mental health.[26] Conversely, negative relationship interactions and low emotional support with social contacts are associated with increased risk of depression.[26] In turn, depression among those with cardiovascular disease or diabetes mellitus is associated with increased risk of substance use, suicidality, and increased mortality.[27–29] These responses to social interactions demonstrate how social engagement may work through different mechanisms, including allostatic load, to affect health outcomes.

NEGATIVE HEALTH CONSEQUENCES OF SOCIAL ISOLATION

Contribution of Isolation to Poor Mental Well-Being

Social isolation, which is the lack of contact with social network members,[30] has negative effects on mental health and well-being across the lifespan. Feelings of loneliness may result from social isolation and is a distinct set of feelings from depression. *Loneliness*, which is the feeling of isolation despite network size and quantity of contacts,[30] has been identified as a significant risk factor for depression among older adults even after consideration of demographics, marital status, social isolation, and other psychosocial risk factors. In addition to increased depression, social isolation and loneliness contribute to dementia and poor life satisfaction.[30]

The COVID-19 pandemic has highlighted new consideration about how social isolation may affect mental health among youth, as well. Although evidence is somewhat mixed, loneliness among children has been found to be associated with depression, but causality is not completely established, as depression may lead to isolation and feelings of loneliness, as well.[31] In the context of enforced isolation due to quarantine, parents have reported that children required mental health services due to disease containment procedures, such as required remote schooling and social distancing, in several different epidemics.[31] Quarantine was associated with increased post-traumatic stress disorder symptoms, acute stress disorder, and grief.[31] Isolation and loneliness during the COVID-19 pandemic was associated with increased anxiety and depression among adolescents.[32] It is possible, however, that increased access to electronic social media, particularly face-to-face contact with friends and family mediated through electronic forums, may buffer the association between isolation and poor mental health outcomes among both adolescents and adults.[33–35]

Effect of Isolation on Physical Health

Social isolation also has deleterious effects on physical health. Social isolation and loneliness have been linked to several negative physical health outcomes, including any-cause mortality, falls, serious psychological illness, faster functional decline, and malnutrition.[30] Family care practitioners are well situated to identifying patients at risk of social isolation and loneliness and helping patients to engage in a way that may improve these issues. Risk factors associated with loneliness and isolation include: older age, female gender, lower income, residence in rural areas, and living in long-term care.[30] In addition, patients who live far from others and who live alone are caregivers to a relative, have had recent major life changes, or who lack transportation may be more likely to experience social isolation and loneliness.

Marital Status and Contribution to Social Isolation

Marital status has long been recognized as an important factor associated with health and mortality among middle-aged and older adults.[36] Married individuals have improved health and lower mortality, particularly among men.[36] Unmarried status is associated with higher risk of mortality from all causes, particularly in those who had never been married.[37] Marriage has a particular advantage for improved mortality among men, however, who have increased risk of early mortality among never married or divorced men compared to women in the same marital status categories.[37] It may be that some of these differences are due to increased social support and engagement that enable them to better buffer stress experiences while men rely more on their wives for social supports and are more isolated across the life course compared to women.[37–39] Further, men who live alone or have poor marital quality may be more likely to avoid health care or be less likely to adhere to their health care provider's advice to improve their health outcomes and have higher levels of loneliness compared to women with similar marital status.[37,40]

Divorce and widowed status also play a role in feelings of loneliness. Individuals who start living alone after divorce or loss of a partner exhibit a higher risk of mortality compared to those who live with others as well as those who lived alone without loss of a partner.[41] Being unmarried has been found to be associated with increased odds of misusing combined opioid and benzodiazepine among older adults, particularly among those who had been divorced or separated or never married.[42] The stress associated with social isolation and loneliness may contribute to self-medication or other unhealthy coping mechanisms to alleviate those feelings.

POSITIVE HEALTH CONSEQUENCES OF SOCIAL CONNECTEDNESS

Social Networks as Systems for Support

Social support is an important contributor to mental health and well-being among diverse populations in the United States. Social support, particularly supportive communication, has been shown to serve as a protective factor for psychological distress among black Americans, Hispanics, Asian Americans, and other marginalized communities.[43–47] Social support makes the effects of loneliness on depression or anxiety smaller by improving an individual's resilience and providing them with socially rewarding roles that improves positivity and life outlook.[48] For example, among patients diagnosed with medically unexplained symptoms, the negative effects of loneliness on anxiety and depression were decreased among those who reported higher social support.[48]

Physicians can contribute to improving their patients' mental and physical health by recommending patients to engage in community-based group classes and through encouraging utilization of social contacts, online communities, and family to help patients develop healthy coping strategies that can buffer the effects of stress and allostatic load on health.[49] Peer-to-peer support groups have been offered to improve social support and related health outcomes. Participation in peer groups, such as 12-step programs, has shown to improve abstinence behaviors, particularly among those who attended more meetings, had more sponsor meetings, and doing service.[50] Having at least 2 or more social network members who abstained as well were long-term predictors of continued abstinence.[50] Peer support systems have also been shown to improve outcomes among individuals with a variety of health conditions to improve health behaviors through improving perceived social support and emotional well-being.[51] Another example is that patients who had weight-loss surgery achieved enhanced adherence to behavioral change and self-management if they attended peer-support weight management sessions facilitated by a social worker and a dietitian compared to those with individual follow-up meetings with dieticians only.[52]

STIGMA AS A BARRIER TO PREVENTION CARE AND TREATMENT ACCESS

Stigma Effects on Mental Well-Being

Stigma, defined as a strong lack of respect or poor opinion for a person or group because of a quality or behavior not acceptable in society, is a powerful social determinant of health that acts as a barrier to access and engagement in the health care system and treatment adherence.[53,54] Stigma in health care stems from a lack of understanding and negative beliefs and attitudes regarding a particular health condition group of people affected by the condition. Experiences of stigma are often reported by people with mental illness. In the United States, over 50% of the population will experience a mental illness during their lifetime, and 1 in 5 will experience a mental illness in any given year. Despite this, only 51.2% of female and 37.4% of male individuals received mental health care in the United States in 2020 due to reasons including the pervasiveness of stigma attached to seeking mental health care.[55] Many myths and stereotypes are associated with mental illness, including that the person is violent, has a character flaw, or that they are unable to take care of themselves. Stereotypes can lead to discriminatory behavior perpetrated upon the individual, often exacerbating mental illness, or serving as a deterrent to seeking care.

Mental health stigma has been associated with social isolation, poverty,[56] housing instability and homelessness,[57] unstable employment,[58] and suicide.[59] Mental health conditions, such as depression, have been correlated with many chronic diseases, including diabetes mellitus, asthma, cancer, and cardiovascular disease.[60] Patients with comorbid mental health and physical health conditions may find it difficult to maintain routine medical appointments or adhere to treatment plans.

Stigma as a Barrier to Treatment

Stigma occurs at several levels and contributes to poor health outcomes. It may affect how a provider communicates with their patients, contributing to suboptimal preventive health care. Stigma from health care providers is positively associated with disempowerment, and may cause reluctance among patients with stigmatized conditions to seek care or continue treatment due to internalized stigma, guilt, or even due to providers withholding care.[61–63] Stigmatizing language used by health care providers may reinforce these stereotypes.

Providers who read vignettes about substance use disorder were more likely to have negative attitudes toward patients if notes referred to them as "substance abusers" as compared to notes that used the term "having a substance use disorder."[64] This is especially concerning as health care providers have been noted to include negative impressions about truthfulness, disapproval of patient decisions or health behaviors, racial or social class stereotypes, individual frustrations, or subjective valuations of patient unreasonableness in encounter notes that could contribute to further stigmatization of patients by themselves or other providers who read those comments in the future.[65] Resources to guide professionals in language to use and avoid are available (**Table 1**).

Interacting with patients in a nonjudgmental way can help to increase their self-efficacy and encourage them to feel confident about continuing to attend future appointments and improve their adherence to their care plan.[66] This in turn improves their health outcomes. It is difficult to quantify ethically the direct effects of reduced stigma on patient health outcomes, but qualitative research has indicated the importance of nonstigmatized care for patients. In a study of the effects of provider stigma among patients with binge-eating disorder, participants described stigmatized interactions with previous health care encounters as having decreased the quality of care they received.[67] In another study of diabetes outcomes among young patients, less stigma in interactions with providers was associated with better control of the condition and less complications.[68]

Stigma manifests in several different forms that interact to create barriers to care. Public stigma is the reaction to another perceived to have a stigmatized condition.

Table 1
Resources to assist providers in avoiding the use of stigmatic language for common conditions

Resource Origin	Purpose	Link	Type
National Institute on Drug Abuse (NIDA)	Terms to avoid when talking about addiction	https://nida.nih.gov/nidamed-medical-health-professionals/health-professions-education/words-matter-terms-to-use-avoid-when-talking-about-addiction	Website
Centers for Disease Control and Prevention (CDC)	Provider stigma about substance use	https://www.cdc.gov/stopoverdose/stigma/index.html	Website
Substance Abuse and Mental Health Services Administration (SAMHSA)	Resource guide: reducing discriminatory practices in clinical settings	https://www.samhsa.gov/sites/default/files/programs_campaigns/02._webcast_3_resources.pdf	PDF
American Hospital Association	Series of downloadable posters to help employees adopt patient-centered, respectful language	https://www.aha.org/people-matter-words-matter	Posters
World Obesity	Examples of language to avoid and adopt when talking about obesity	https://www.worldobesity.org/downloads/healthy_voices_downloads/HV_Language_guidelines.pdf	PDF
Obesity Action Coalition	Provide examples of people-first language to reduce stigma	https://www.obesityaction.org/action-through-advocacy/weight-bias/people-first-language/	Website
	Addresses provider stigma	https://www.obesityaction.org/get-educated/public-resources/brochures-guides/understanding-obesity-stigma-brochure/	Brochure
MentalHealthyFit	Videos to make sense of mental health through film	https://mentalhealthyfit.org/films?gclid=CjwKCAjwzuqgBhAcEiwAdj5dRpWKyBVBgTRUD6u69Ez-sYdIA-JIDtQHoOCZmrIzXwFEYpV-PWruVhoCiMUQAvD_BwE	Website with video

(*continued on next page*)

Table 1
(*continued*)

Resource Origin	Purpose	Link	Type
National Council for Mental Wellbeing	Training to use person-first language to create more inclusive language in discussions about mental health	https://www.mentalhealthfirstaid.org/2022/04/use-person-first-language-to-reduce-stigma/	Training
The Well Project	Understand stigmatic language surrounding HIV that prevents effective screening and treatment among women	https://www.thewellproject.org/hiv-information/why-language-matters-facing-hiv-stigma-our-own-words	Slide presentation and website
TargetHIV	Reduce provider stigma related to HIV	https://targethiv.org/escalate	Website
National Institute of Allergy and Infectious Diseases (NIAID)	HIV Language Guide	https://www.hptn.org/sites/default/files/inline-files/NIAID%20HIV%20Language%20Guide%20-%20March%202020.pdf	PDF

Self-stigma encompasses an individual's social and psychological effects of having a stigmatized condition. Stigma by association includes the reactions of people to those who are associated to someone with a stigmatized condition, whereas structural stigma includes institutional perpetuations of stigma through legitimizing and perpetuating the reactions to stigma. Although addressing public stigma within the community is important, addressing both structural and public stigma in health care institutions and among providers who refer and treat individuals with stigmatized conditions is critical to improving knowledge and health outcomes.[69] Higher level structural stigmas may affect entire populations, such as exclusionary laws and policies, while other structural stigmas exist that may specifically affect the relationship between a provider and their patient.[70]

Increasing awareness of stigma, engaging in programs to improve provider–patient interactions, and encouraging community awareness of health conditions can decrease stigmatic interactions in both health care and community. Connections between policy-makers, community leaders, and those knowledgeable about stigmatized conditions and the needs surrounding those health issues may improve structural stigma. For example, helping policy makers understand the harmful effects of policy requiring reporting, removing parental rights, and criminalization of pregnant women who consume alcohol on help seeking and treatment can help to reduce stigma and improve supportive policy that focuses on early intervention and treatment.[71]

Structural stigmas that directly affect communication between a patient and health provider include a lack of privacy due to physical settings or communication practices, or limitations in service availability. Patients who observe that their conversations may be heard through the wall, or who hear providers talking about other patients, may feel that their conversations or private information will not be private if shared. It is important that these structural factors be identified and addressed to improve the relationship between health care provider and patient that can contribute to earlier and more effective interventions to promote overall health.

UTILIZATION OF SOCIAL NETWORKS AS A SYSTEM FOR CHANGE

Social Cohesion Effects on Prevention and Treatment of Poor Health

Social cohesion, the sense of belongingness and trust shared by members of society, has been positively associated with many health outcomes, including obesity, depression, and cardiovascular disease.[72–74] Further, social cohesion has had positive impacts on preventive care, such as obtaining vaccinations and screening tests (eg, mammography and prostate cancer screening).[75] Social cohesion is built through a shared commitment to common goals identified by the community and aims to decrease income inequality which has been tied to increased rates of morbidity and mortality. Perceived neighborhood social cohesion has been associated with a lower risk of stroke[76] and lower levels of depression among vulnerable groups such as single mothers, older adults, and adolescents.[77–79]

In recent years, the erosion of social cohesion has been a concern. As gentrification becomes more common in urban areas, communities may see positive effects such as a reduction in poverty and reduced crime. On the other hand, residents who are displaced often experience increased stress, possibly contributing to poor health outcomes especially among Black and low-income individuals.[80]

Primary care providers (PCPs) have long played a pivotal role in addressing mental health concerns and many are comfortable identifying and managing anxiety and depression.[81] Approaching mental health screening from a social determinants of health perspective means that aspects of the patient's social environment that may serve as protective factors must be explored.

Utilizing Community Coalitions and Other Community Resources to Achieve Improved Health

Community coalitions have been instrumental in bringing about change in local communities for well over 5 decades. Coalitions can help bring communities together and improve population health. Rather than focus on the behavior of individuals, research has shown that health promotion must also include intervention at the macro level. By their very nature, coalitions help to promote unity around a shared purpose thus positively contributing to social cohesion. Efforts by community coalitions have contributed to adolescent substance use reduction,[82] dramatic gains in the prevention and control of tobacco use,[83] and reduction in the negative health impact of many chronic diseases, including type II diabetes.[84]

Religion as Support to Engage in Healthy Behavior

Although church membership has seen a gradual decline in the United States since the turn of the century, churches continue to be a strong source of social support for over one-half of the population.[85] Ethnically and racially diverse communities often rely on the church for more than their spiritual needs. For example, in Black communities, residents may feel more comfortable accessing health services within the church, or endorsed by the church, due to the historical mistrust held toward traditional health care settings.[86] Recent literature has suggested that faith-based partnerships can have a positive effect on hypertension and cardiovascular disease.[87] Churches provide a space for gathering and often host health-promotion activities such as cooking classes, health fairs, and mental health services. Many religions also promote healthier lifestyles by following certain dietary laws, such as avoiding certain meats, adopting plant-based diets, and avoiding alcohol.

DISCUSSION

The Role of the Primary Care Provider

Addressing prevention and treatment among socially isolated patients or those with poor social supports

PCPs continually navigate the barriers faced by their patients and seek solutions among local services available, their living environment, and in their social network. The role of the PCP begins with an understanding of the common barriers and resources in the community, then by assessing and responding to the patient's own challenges, and finally by advocating in the clinic and public for changes to the underlying social and structural causes of morbidity and mortality.

Social connectedness is a key component of allostatic load and is considered a significant risk factor for cardiometabolic disease.[3] The high relative importance of social context among modifiable risk factors for chronic physical and mental health problems means the PCP should assess their patients' level of social support and connectedness and encourage participation in support groups and community social activities. Social isolation has long been a focus of research and senior care, but has dramatically grown as a concern for all ages since 2020, as COVID-19 has commonly been described as a "double pandemic" due to isolation, interrupted access to care, and the many other downstream effects.[88] Evidence suggests that all causes of morbidity and mortality are impacted by social connection and are thus an undeniable concern of the PCP.[89,90] Social groups reinforce both good and bad health behaviors, but inclusion in a social group is generally understood to be highly beneficial and especially relevant to the PCP in the treatment adherence domain.[91,92]

PCPs are expanding their range of practice regarding the social determinants of health in recent years, but this improvement is not yet universally applied as a standard of care.[93] Although there may be a limited number of standard ways that the PCP can change the social lives and social determinants of their patients in the clinical encounter, there are subtle practices that can have a significant impact on outcomes. Even minor improvements in communication about the patient's social context and social determinants, such as asking questions about social support and offering resources for isolated patients, can effectively interrupt the cycle of worsening physical and mental state undermining the ability to secure housing, employment, food, social support, and health care. Better outcomes result when almost any communication improvement strategies are employed.[94] Essentially, patients may not fully understand the important takeaways from a clinical encounter, gravely undermining the value of the visit. Many patients report not being asked about their social determinants of health and this may lead to serious missed opportunities and even inappropriate care plans. Asking patients the right questions in a sensitive way establishes knowledge of their situation and trust. Knowing the life challenges facing a patient can make a big difference in the approach to treatment and management. If unable to provide social support resources, understanding of a patient's situation will at least allow for modification of the treatment plan in some cases to enable better patient adherence to the care plan.

The patient's environment and social/familial circumstances are largely beyond the control of the PCP, but there are often opportunities for the PCP to either exacerbate or ameliorate the situation, and it is in this marginal difference where gains can be made. Issues like ability to afford medications and food, intimate partner violence, or substance use are clear examples where the primary care physician awareness can affect the care plan significantly, and social support should be included in this assessment as it can be the key barrier or resolution.[95] For example, it is important for the PCP to evaluate the efficacy of medication or behavior change in the context of the patient's relative ease or difficulty with treatment adherence. It may not be enough, for example, to assume a prescription or referral is sufficient without first establishing the likelihood and feasibility of adherence.[96]

If adherence is unlikely, then additional time and personnel should be dedicated to finding solutions. A supportive family member or friend can make the difference when transportation or medication adherence is difficult. The PCP must also consider stigma as a functional limit on what information the patient is willing to share; however, standardized and self-administered screening tools and algorithms can help to reduce hesitance to respond and reduce variability in practitioner unconscious bias.

Navigation of the disparities and stigma surrounding mental and preventive health care among racial/ethnic minorities

Health care providers must address and overcome stigma surrounding health topics that affect their patients' health. To provide unbiased care that decreases disparities surrounding topics such as substance use, obesity, sexually transmitted infections, and many others, providers must recognize and overcome their implicit and explicit biases.[97] Health care providers may seek additional training and resources relating to care for patients with stigmatized conditions in states or for conditions for which it is not mandated. Multiple resources on addressing provider stigma for different health conditions are available through a variety of organizations such as through the Obesity Action Coalition, the Centers for Disease Control and Prevention for substance use, and TargetHIV among others (see **Table 1**).

Table 2
Resources to assist providers in screening for social determinants of health

Resource Origin	Name of Tool	Link	Type
American Academy of Family Physicians (AAFP)	Core Social Needs screening tool	https://www.aafp.org/dam/AAFP/documents/patient_care/everyone_project/hops19-physician-form-sdoh.pdf	PDF
Centers for Medicare and Medicaid Services (CMS)	Accountable Health Communities (AHC) Health-Related Social Needs (HRSN) screening tool	https://innovation.cms.gov/files/worksheets/ahcm-screeningtool.pdf	PDF
American Academy of Family Physicians (AAFP)	AAFP Neighborhood Navigator to identify local barriers and resources	https://www.aafp.org/dam/AAFP/documents/patient_care/everyone_project/hops19-physician-guide-sdoh.pdf	PDF
American Academy of Family Physicians (AAFP)	Patient Action Plan	https://www.aafp.org/dam/AAFP/documents/patient_care/everyone_project/action-plan.pdf	PDF
American Academy of Family Physicians (AAFP)	Snapshot of community social determinants of health	https://www.aafp.org/dam/AAFP/documents/patient_care/everyone_project/action-plan.pdf	PDF
County Health Rankings & Roadmaps		www.countyhealthrankings.org	Website

Leveraging community and social resources to improve prevention and treatment outcomes

The American Academy of Family Physicians (AAFP) offers a brief 15-question "Core Social Needs" screening tool that evaluates basic measures for the social determinants with the greatest impact on health, that are potentially addressable, but are often not addressed. These factors include instability in housing, food, transport, utilities, childcare, employment, education, finances, and personal safety. They note that not all factors surveyed must be addressed in one visit, and not solely by the physician either, but rather longitudinally and in coordination with the rest of the health care team. Although they recommend a team-based approach to practice use of the measure with roles for each team member, they acknowledge this is not always feasible as all practices are different in structure as are the community resources available. Of note, absent from this questionnaire are direct questions about social support, so some additional discussion may be required. Alternatively, Centers for Medicare & Medicaid Services (CMS) have a similar but longer-form screening tool available that includes social support questions (**Table 2**).

In light of the variability of populations, environments, and resources available, AAFP also recommends some tools for providers to learn more about their local barriers and resources including the AAFP Neighborhood Navigator, which helps identify local social services, the Patient Action Plan helps to identify referrals needed, and County Health Rankings & Roadmaps, which provides a snapshot of community social determinants of health.

Another role of the PCP is the appropriate referral to social work agencies, support groups, behavioral health, and community organizations that may provide help in and beyond the clinical visit. Some key examples of such resource linkages that may seem to go above and beyond the role of the PCP but are increasingly recommended solutions include clinical partnerships with public service agencies for housing and employment and even legal aid workers.[93]

Much work to date on this subject concludes that PCPs must advocate for improving the underlying social context, behavioral and social aspects of care, not only on a per-patient basis, but at the practice and community levels. This means leading the culture change toward holistic team-based care in the workplace and advocating for patients' environmental and service availability needs in civil society and policymaking.[95] The PCP is charged with this public advocacy partly due to their intimate and privileged understanding of the true needs of their patients and community. They are also the most trusted authority on health and retain the ability to promote truthful narratives to counteract the untrue conventional wisdom and disinformation available.[98]

CLINICS CARE POINTS

- PCPs should consider their patients' social and behavioral factors during clinical visits, with awareness that social circumstances may change between visits. Careful questioning and use of special tools, including surveys, for this purpose are freely available and can help the clinician decide with the patient what care would best fit their circumstances.
- When encountering a patient with a stigmatized condition, including mental health conditions, health care providers should avoid stigmatizing language. Awareness of language use and training that is focused on reducing stigma in health care is widely available through online sources.

- Screening for social engagement and support will help the clinician to better understand the environment the patient is surrounded by. This awareness allows the clinician to adjust care plans, particularly for mental health conditions or substance use, that the patient encounters in their daily activities. It will also help the provider better understand the need for peer counseling or other programs that can assist the patient to accumulate more resources to improve their resilience and achieve improved outcomes.
- Social isolation and loneliness are particularly detrimental to mental and physical health. PCPs can improve their communication surrounding these issues so they may offer appropriate resources to improve health outcomes through reducing missed opportunities and increasing the ability to modify treatment plans that encourage better patient adherence.

FUNDING

JMH: National Research Service Award in Primary Care (T32 training grant) - #T32 HP10031, Project REACH: Improve HIV and Hepatitis C prevention, screening and access to recovery services for individuals with a substance use disorder and/or co-occurring substance use and mental health disorders - #TI080624-01(09/30/2018 - 09/29/2023) Grant funding from SAMHSA, Bringing Alcohol and Other Drug Research to Primary Care - #1R25AA028203-01$664,777.00 (04/01/2020 - 03/31/2024)Grant funding from NIAAA. SJG: SM081472 SAMHSA Gonzalez (PD) 04/30/2020 – 04/29/2023Mental Health Awareness Training – Aware HoustonRole: PI/Project DirectorTI082637 SAMHSA Zoorob (PD) 04/30/2020 – 04/29/2025 Grants for the Benefit of Homeless Individuals – Come Home HoustonRole: Evaluator 1R25AA028203 NIH/NIAAA Zoorob/Kowalchuk (MPI) 04/01/2020 – 03/31/2024Bringing Alcohol and Other Drug Research to Primary CareRole: Co-Investigator U01-DD001131 CDC Zoorob (PI/PD) 09/2014 – 09/2018Fetal Alcohol Spectrum Disorders Practice and Implementation Centers Role: Co-Investigator, Content Expert for Social Work. RZ: Equitable Access to Lung Cancer Screening and Smoking Cessation Treatment: A Comprehensive Primary Care and Community Health Approach - #PP180016(03/01/2018 - 02/28/2021) Grant funding from Cancer Prevention and Research Institute of Texas (CPRIT)National Research Service Award in Primary Care (T32 training grant) - #T32 HP10031$1,725,796.00 (07/01/2016 - 05/30/2021) Grant funding from HRSAProject REACH: Improve HIV and Hepatitis C prevention, screening and access to recovery services for individuals with a substance use disorder and/or co-occurring substance use and mental health disorders - #TI080624-01(09/30/2018 - 09/29/2023) Grant funding from SAMHSABaylor College of Medicine Center of Excellence in Health Equity, Training, and Research - #D34HP31024(07/01/2017 - 06/01/2022) Grant funding from HRSABringing Alcohol and Other Drug Research to Primary Care - #1R25AA028203-01$664,777.00 (04/01/2020 - 03/31/2024)Grant funding from NIAAAAWARE-HOUSTON - #SM081472$347,164.00 (04/30/2020 - 04/29/2023)Grant funding from MHAT/SAMHSACome Home Houston - #1H79TI082637-01$399,275.00 (04/30/2020 - 04/29/2025)Grant funding from SAMHSAEquitable Access to Lung Cancer Screening and Smoking Cessation Treatment: A Comprehensive Primary Care and Community Health Approach - #PP180016(03/01/2018 - 02/28/2021) Grant funding from Cancer Prevention and Research Institute of TexasProject Reach: Improve HIV and Hepatitis C Prevention, Screening and Access to Recovery Services for Individuals with a Substance Use Disorder and/or Co-occurring Substance Use and Mental Health Disorders - #TI080624-01$500,000.00 (09/30/2018 - 09/29/2023)Grant funding from SAMHSA.

DISCLOSURE

The authors have nothing to disclose.

REFERENCES

1. Umberson D, Karas Montez J. Social Relationships and Health: A Flashpoint for Health Policy. J Health Soc Behav 2010;51(1_suppl):S54–66.
2. Carbone JT, Clift J, Alexander N. Measuring allostatic load: Approaches and limitations to algorithm creation. J Psychosom Res 2022;163:111050.
3. Guidi J, Lucente M, Sonino N, et al. Allostatic Load and Its Impact on Health: A Systematic Review. Psychother Psychosom 2021;90(1):11–27.
4. A definition of "social environment. Am J Publ Health 2001;91(3):465a.
5. Maghsoudi Z, Sadeghi A, Oshvandi K, et al. Barriers to Treatment Adherence Among Older Adults With Type 2 Diabetes: A Qualitative Study. J Gerontol Nurs 2023;49(1):42–9.
6. Stephen G, Muldoon Orla T, Bennett Kate M. Multiple group membership, social network size, allostatic load and well-being: A mediation analysis. J Psychosom Res 2021;151:110636.
7. Cofie LE, Hirth JM, Lee JGL. Social Support Networks and Foreign-Birth Status Associated With Obesity, Hypertension and Diabetes Prevalence Among 21-30 and 50-70 Year Old Adults Living in the San Francisco Bay Area. Am J Health Promot 2021;35(8):1105–13.
8. Larson NI, Wall MM, Story MT, et al. Home/family, peer, school, and neighborhood correlates of obesity in adolescents. Obesity 2013;21(9):1858–69.
9. Berkman LF. Assessing the physical health effects of social networks and social support. Annu Rev Publ Health 1984;5(1):413–32.
10. Thoits PA. Mechanisms linking social ties and support to physical and mental health. J Health Soc Behav 2011;52(2):145–61.
11. Christakis NA, Fowler JH. The spread of obesity in a large social network over 32 years. N Engl J Med 2007;357(4):370–9.
12. Havassy BE, Hall SM, Wasserman DA. Social support and relapse: commonalities among alcoholics, opiate users, and cigarette smokers. Addict Behav 1991;16(5):235–46.
13. Marroni CA, Fleck AM Jr, Fernandes SA, et al. Liver transplantation and alcoholic liver disease: History, controversies, and considerations. World J Gastroenterol 2018;24(26):2785–805.
14. Hutchison C. Social support: factors to consider when designing studies that measure social support. J Adv Nurs 1999;29(6):1520–6.
15. Rieger E, Sellbom M, Murray K, et al. Measuring social support for healthy eating and physical activity in obesity. Br J Health Psychol 2018;23(4):1021–39.
16. Krause N, Markides K. Measuring social support among older adults. Int J Aging Hum Dev 1990;30(1):37–53.
17. Heitzmann CA, Kaplan RM. Assessment of methods for measuring social support. Health Psychol 1988;7(1):75–109.
18. Kim ES, Whillans AV, Lee MT, et al. Volunteering and Subsequent Health and Well-Being in Older Adults: An Outcome-Wide Longitudinal Approach. Am J Prev Med 2020;59(2):176–86.
19. Carson AP, Rose KM, Catellier DJ, et al. Employment Status, Coronary Heart Disease, and Stroke Among Women. Ann Epidemiol 2009;19(9):630–6.
20. Harrison AS, Sumner J, McMillan D, et al. Relationship between employment and mental health outcomes following Cardiac Rehabilitation: an observational

analysis from the National Audit of Cardiac Rehabilitation. Int J Cardiol 2016;220: 851–4.
21. Bath PA, Deeg D. Social engagement and health outcomes among older people: introduction to a special section. Eur J Ageing 2005;2(1):24–30.
22. Majoka MA, Schimming C. Effect of Social Determinants of Health on Cognition and Risk of Alzheimer Disease and Related Dementias. Clin Therapeut 2021; 43(6):922–9.
23. Mishra SK, Togneri E, Tripathi B, et al. Spirituality and Religiosity and Its Role in Health and Diseases. J Relig Health 2017;56(4):1282–301.
24. Castagné R, Garès V, Karimi M, et al. Allostatic load and subsequent all-cause mortality: which biological markers drive the relationship? Findings from a UK birth cohort. Eur J Epidemiol 2018;33(5):441–58.
25. Fiksdal A, Hanlin L, Kuras Y, et al. Associations between symptoms of depression and anxiety and cortisol responses to and recovery from acute stress. Psychoneuroendocrinology 2019;102:44–52.
26. Sarris J, O'Neil A, Coulson CE, et al. Lifestyle medicine for depression. BMC Psychiatr 2014;14(1):107.
27. Davis L, Uezato A, Newell JM, et al. Major depression and comorbid substance use disorders. Curr Opin Psychiatry 2008;21(1):14–8.
28. Tirado Muñoz J, Farré A, Mestre-Pintó J, et al. Patología dual en Depresión: recomendaciones en el tratamiento. Adicciones 2017;30(1):66.
29. Goldstein CM, Gathright EC, Garcia S. Relationship between depression and medication adherence in cardiovascular disease: the perfect challenge for the integrated care team. Patient Prefer Adherence 2017;11:547–59.
30. Freedman A, Nicolle J. Social isolation and loneliness: the new geriatric giants: Approach for primary care. Can Fam Physician 2020;66(3):176–82.
31. Loades ME, Chatburn E, Higson-Sweeney N, et al. Rapid Systematic Review: The Impact of Social Isolation and Loneliness on the Mental Health of Children and Adolescents in the Context of COVID-19. J Am Acad Child Adolesc Psychiatr 2020;59(11):1218–39.e3.
32. Meade J. Mental Health Effects of the COVID-19 Pandemic on Children and Adolescents: A Review of the Current Research. Pediatr Clin North Am 2021;68(5): 945–59.
33. Orben A, Tomova L, Blakemore S-J. The effects of social deprivation on adolescent development and mental health. The Lancet Child & Adolescent Health 2020;4(8):634–40.
34. Saltzman LY, Hansel TC, Bordnick PS. Loneliness, isolation, and social support factors in post-COVID-19 mental health. Psychol Trauma 2020;12(S1):S55–s57.
35. Cosco TD, Fortuna K, Wister A, et al. COVID-19, Social Isolation, and Mental Health Among Older Adults: A Digital Catch-22. J Med Internet Res 2021; 23(5):e21864.
36. Robards J, Evandrou M, Falkingham J, et al. Marital status, health and mortality. Maturitas 2012;73(4):295–9.
37. Wang Y, Jiao Y, Nie J, et al. Sex differences in the association between marital status and the risk of cardiovascular, cancer, and all-cause mortality: a systematic review and meta-analysis of 7,881,040 individuals. Global Health Research and Policy 2020;5(1):4.
38. Simon H. Marriage and men's health. Harv Mens Health Watch 2010;14(12):1–5.
39. Umberson D, Lin Z, Cha H. Gender and Social Isolation across the Life Course. J Health Soc Behav 2022;63(3):319–35.

40. Dafoe WA, Colella TJ. Loneliness, marriage and cardiovascular health. Eur J Prev Cardiol 2016;23(12):1242–4.
41. Abell JG, Steptoe A. Why is living alone in older age related to increased mortality risk? A longitudinal cohort study. Age Ageing 2021;50(6):2019–24.
42. Day BF, Rosenthal GL. Social isolation proxy variables and prescription opioid and benzodiazepine misuse among older adults in the U.S.: A cross-sectional analysis of data from the National Survey on Drug Use and Health, 2015-2017. Drug Alcohol Depend 2019;204:107518.
43. Steers MN, Chen TA, Neisler J, et al. The buffering effect of social support on the relationship between discrimination and psychological distress among church-going African-American adults. Behav Res Ther 2019;115:121–8.
44. Guntzviller LM, Williamson LD, Ratcliff CL. Stress, Social Support, and Mental Health Among Young Adult Hispanics. Fam Community Health 2020;43(1):82–91.
45. Griffith J. Emotional support providers and psychological distress among Anglo- and Mexican Americans. Community Ment Health J 1984;20(3):182–201.
46. Zhang L, Cruz-Gonzalez M, Lin Z, et al. Association of everyday discrimination with health outcomes among Asian and non-Asian US older adults before and during the COVID-19 pandemic. Front Public Health 2022;10:953155.
47. McDonald K. Social Support and Mental Health in LGBTQ Adolescents: A review of the literature. Issues Ment Health Nurs 2018;39(1):16–29.
48. Hutten E, Jongen EMM, Vos A, et al. Loneliness and Mental Health: The Mediating Effect of Perceived Social Support. Int J Environ Res Public Health 2021; 18(22). https://doi.org/10.3390/ijerph182211963.
49. McDaniels B, Pontone GM, Keener AM, et al. A Prescription for Wellness in Early PD: Just What the Doctor Ordered. J Geriatr Psychiatr Neurol 2023. https://doi.org/10.1177/08919887231164358. 08919887231164358.
50. Witbrodt J, Kaskutas LA. Does diagnosis matter? Differential effects of 12-step participation and social networks on abstinence. Am J Drug Alcohol Abuse 2005;31(4):685–707.
51. Hogan BE, Linden W, Najarian B. Social support interventions: do they work? Clin Psychol Rev 2002;22(3):383–442.
52. Shinan-Altman S, Sandbank GK, Natarevich-Katzav H, et al. Self-management After Bariatric Surgery: a Comparison Between Support Group Participants and Patients Receiving Individual Dietary Follow-Up. Obes Surg 2023;33(3):826–35.
53. Knaak S, Mantler E, Szeto A. Mental illness-related stigma in healthcare. Healthc Manag Forum 2017;30(2):111–6.
54. Katz IT, Ryu AE, Onuegbu AG, et al. Impact of HIV-related stigma on treatment adherence: systematic review and meta-synthesis. J Int AIDS Soc 2013; 16(Suppl 2):18640.
55. Substance Abuse and Mental Health Services Administration (SAMHSA). 2020 NSDUH Annual National Report. 2021. Annual Report. Oct 25. Available at: https://www.samhsa.gov/data/report/2020-nsduh-annual-national-report. Accessed March 23, 2023.
56. Knifton L, Inglis G. Poverty and mental health: policy, practice and research implications. BJPsych Bull 2020;44(5):193–6.
57. Mejia-Lancheros C, Lachaud J, O'Campo P, et al. Trajectories and mental health-related predictors of perceived discrimination and stigma among homeless adults with mental illness. PLoS One 2020;15(2):e0229385.
58. Brouwers EPM. Social stigma is an underestimated contributing factor to unemployment in people with mental illness or mental health issues: position paper and future directions. BMC Psychol 2020;8(1):36.

59. Scocco P, Preti A, Totaro S, et al. Stigma and psychological distress in suicide survivors. J Psychosom Res 2017;94:39–46.
60. Birk JL, Kronish IM, Moise N, et al. Depression and multimorbidity: Considering temporal characteristics of the associations between depression and multiple chronic diseases. Health Psychol 2019;38(9):802–11.
61. Dubin RE, Kaplan A, Graves L, et al. Acknowledging stigma: Its presence in patient care and medical education. Can Fam Physician 2017;63(12):906–8.
62. Wang K, Link BG, Corrigan PW, et al. Perceived provider stigma as a predictor of mental health service users' internalized stigma and disempowerment. Psychiatr Res 2018;259:526–31.
63. Carol M, Pérez-Guasch M, Solà E, et al. Stigmatization is common in patients with non-alcoholic fatty liver disease and correlates with quality of life. PLoS One 2022; 17(4):e0265153.
64. Kelly JF, Westerhoff CM. Does it matter how we refer to individuals with substance-related conditions? A randomized study of two commonly used terms. Int J Drug Pol 2010;21(3):202–7.
65. Park J, Saha S, Chee B, et al. Physician Use of Stigmatizing Language in Patient Medical Records. JAMA Netw Open 2021;4(7):e2117052.
66. Chan B, Geduldig A, Korthuis T, et al. The SUMMIT Team is All I Got": perspectives of medically and socially complex patients seen in intensive primary care. Ann Fam Med 2022;(20 Suppl 1). https://doi.org/10.1370/afm.20.s1.3043.
67. Salvia MG, Ritholz MD, Craigen KLE, et al. Women's perceptions of weight stigma and experiences of weight-neutral treatment for binge eating disorder: A qualitative study. EClinicalMedicine 2023;56:101811.
68. Eitel KB, Roberts AJ, D'Agostino R, et al. Diabetes Stigma and Clinical Outcomes in Adolescents and Young Adults: the SEARCH for Diabetes in Youth Study. Diabetes Care 2023. https://doi.org/10.2337/dc22-1749.
69. Bos AER, Pryor JB, Reeder GD, et al. Stigma: Advances in theory and research. Basic Appl Soc Psychol 2013;35:1–9.
70. Bolster-Foucault C, Ho Mi Fane B, Blair A. Structural determinants of stigma across health and social conditions: a rapid review and conceptual framework to guide future research and intervention. Health Promot Chronic Dis Prev Can 2021;41(3):85–115. Déterminants structurels de la stigmatisation touchant les conditions sanitaires et sociales : revue rapide et cadre conceptuel visant à guider la recherche et les interventions.
71. Roozen S, Stutterheim SE, Bos AER, et al. Understanding the Social Stigma of Fetal Alcohol Spectrum Disorders: From Theory to Interventions. Found Sci 2022;27(2):753–71.
72. Cuevas AG, Kawachi I, Ortiz K, et al. Greater social cohesion is associated with lower body mass index among African American adults. Preventive Medicine Reports 2020;18:101098.
73. Perez LG, Arredondo EM, McKenzie TL, et al. Neighborhood Social Cohesion and Depressive Symptoms Among Latinos: Does Use of Community Resources for Physical Activity Matter? J Phys Act Health 2015;12(10):1361–8.
74. Singh R, Javed Z, Yahya T, et al. Community and Social Context: An Important Social Determinant of Cardiovascular Disease. Methodist Debakey Cardiovasc J 2021;17(4):15–27.
75. Kim ES, Kawachi I. Perceived Neighborhood Social Cohesion and Preventive Healthcare Use. Am J Prev Med 2017;53(2):e35–40.
76. Kim ES, Park N, Peterson C. Perceived neighborhood social cohesion and stroke. Soc Sci Med 2013;97:49–55.

77. Fagan AA, Wright EM, Pinchevsky GM. The protective effects of neighborhood collective efficacy on adolescent substance use and violence following exposure to violence. J Youth Adolesc 2014;43(9):1498–512.
78. Barnhart S, Maguire-Jack K. Single mothers in their communities: the mediating role of parenting stress and depression between social cohesion, social control and child maltreatment. Child Youth Serv Rev 2016;70:37–45.
79. Pabayo R, Dunn EC, Gilman SE, et al. Income inequality within urban settings and depressive symptoms among adolescents. J Epidemiol Community Health 2016; 70(10):997–1003.
80. Smith GS, Breakstone H, Dean LT, et al. Impacts of Gentrification on Health in the US: a Systematic Review of the Literature. J Urban Health 2020;97(6):845–56.
81. Collins KA, Wolfe VV, Fisman S, et al. Managing depression in primary care: community survey. Can Fam Physician 2006;52(7):878–9.
82. Hutchison M, Russell BS. Community Coalition Efforts to Prevent Adolescent Substance Use: A Systematic Review. J Drug Educ 2021;50(1–2):3–30.
83. Fallin A, Glantz SA. Tobacco-control policies in tobacco-growing states: where tobacco was king. Milbank Q 2015;93(2):319–58.
84. Janosky JE, Armoutliev EM, Benipal A, et al. Coalitions for impacting the health of a community: the Summit County, Ohio, experience. Popul Health Manag 2013; 16(4):246–54.
85. U.S. Church Membership Falls Below Majority for First Time. Gallup; March 29, 2021. Available at: https://news.gallup.com/poll/341963/church-membership-falls-below-majority-first-time.aspx Accessed March 23, 2023.
86. Giger JN, Appel SJ, Davidhizar R, et al. Church and spirituality in the lives of the African American community. J Transcult Nurs 2008;19(4):375–83.
87. Ferdinand DP, Nedunchezhian S, Ferdinand KC. Hypertension in African Americans: Advances in community outreach and public health approaches. Prog Cardiovasc Dis 2020;63(1):40–5.
88. Galvez-Hernandez P, González-De Paz L, Muntaner C. Primary care-based interventions addressing social isolation and loneliness in older people: a scoping review. BMJ Open 2022;12(2):e057729.
89. Social Isolation And Health, Health Affairs Health Policy Brief, June 21, 2020. https://doi.org/10.1377/hpb20200622.253235.
90. Pantell M, Rehkopf D, Jutte D, et al. Social Isolation: A Predictor of Mortality Comparable to Traditional Clinical Risk Factors. Am J Publ Health 2013;103(11): 2056–62.
91. Larrabee Sonderlund A, Thilsing T, Sondergaard J. Should social disconnectedness be included in primary-care screening for cardiometabolic disease? A systematic review of the relationship between everyday stress, social connectedness, and allostatic load. PLoS One 2019;14(12):e0226717.
92. Wilder ME, Kulie P, Jensen C, et al. The Impact of Social Determinants of Health on Medication Adherence: a Systematic Review and Meta-analysis. J Gen Intern Med 2021;36(5):1359–70.
93. Bloch G, Rozmovits L. Implementing social interventions in primary care. Can Med Assoc J 2021;193(44):E1696–701.
94. Lie HC, Juvet LK, Street RL, et al. Effects of Physicians' Information Giving on Patient Outcomes: a Systematic Review. J Gen Intern Med 2022;37(3):651–63.
95. Andermann A. Taking action on the social determinants of health in clinical practice: a framework for health professionals. Can Med Assoc J 2016;188(17–18): E474–83.

96. Dulin M. What primary care physicians need to know about social determinants of health. In: Medical Economics, editor. Medical Economics2021. Available at: https://www.medicaleconomics.com/view/what-primary-care-physicians-need-to-know-about-social-determinants-of-health.
97. Fruh SM, Nadglowski J, Hall HR, et al. Obesity Stigma and Bias. J Nurse Pract 2016;12(7):425–32.
98. Maani N, Galea S. The Role of Physicians in Addressing Social Determinants of Health. JAMA 2020;323(16):1551.

The Work, Play, and Worship Environments as Social Determinants of Health

Heather M. O'Hara, MD, MPH

KEYWORDS

- SDOH • Social determinants of health • Worship and patient health
- Patient spirituality in primary care clinic • Workers' health and primary care visits
- Social interactions and health

KEY POINTS

- Work, play, and worship in healthcare is paramount to being able to gain traction on improving health and reducing poor outcomes in any population.
- Incorporation of SDOH cannot occur in a silo and utilization of multidisciplinary treatment plans is crucial to being successful.
- Review of and partnership with the resources available in the communities served provides the ability to offer more holistic care.
- Primary care providers have a key role in providing guidance to patients that will help them start or locate support systems for their nonmedical needs.
- Development of a system to direct patient and community care towards various support systems is crucial to decreasing the negative effects of unmet social determinants of health.

INTRODUCTION

Many sectors of health care have long included social determinants of health (SDOHs) as considerations in their practice.[1–3] Understanding and including aspects of access to health care, economic stability and the environmental surroundings as part of the treatment plan provides a holistic approach to improving the health of patients and communities. Although there may be a lack of awareness as to the overarching concept of these areas, the SDOHs include situations and experiences that shape a person or community from conception to death. Reflecting on the interconnection of nonmedical factors that contribute to health is understood to be an important component to achieving overall improvement in health and prevention of various medical illnesses and life decisions.[4] According to *Healthy People 2030*, 5 domains

Memorial Occupational Health Clinic, 2120 North 27th Street, Decatur, IL 62526, USA
E-mail address: Ohara.heather@mhsil.com

Prim Care Clin Office Pract 50 (2023) 621–631
https://doi.org/10.1016/j.pop.2023.04.009
primarycare.theclinics.com

encompass the full range of social interactions that can affect one's health (**Fig. 1**). It is reported that while approximately 20% of health is due to clinical treatment, another 50% to 80% is made up of factors from these domains.[5] Consideration of these domains in health care is paramount to being able to gain traction on improving health and reducing poor outcomes in any population. Areas of life that can be directly linked to one or more of the domains provided include a person's work, play, and worship activities.

Work is not just about what someone does but where and how they get it done. Physical and chemical hazards have been a long-standing concern for workplace environments.[6] However, there is a wide array of other exposures in the workplace that can affect a worker's health and be linked to the SDOH domains too. These can include exposures to poor working conditions, as well as mental health factors stemming from workplace treatment, or even inadequate resources for workers due to compensation inequalities.[7–9] Another element to consider is the generational effects that occur in families that live in poverty despite being employed and how this increases the likelihood of continued poverty for the children that grew up in these

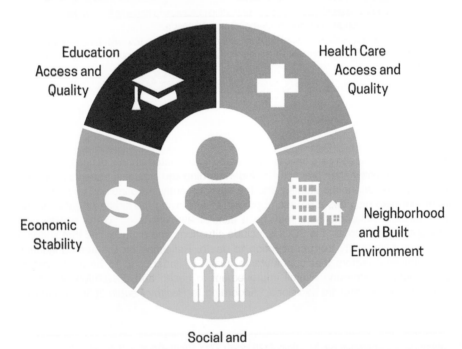

Fig. 1. The 5 domains of the SDOHs. (*From* Healthy People 2030, U.S. Department of Health and Human Services, Office of Disease Prevention and Health Promotion. Accessed October 18, 2022. https://health.gov/healthypeople/objectives-and-data/social-determinants-health.)

situations.[10] Considerations for how these, potentially multifactorial, areas factor into the overall health of workers and communities will help with improving the health dynamic.

The perception of play includes activities that stem from hobbies, leisure or relaxation interests, community partnerships, or even participation in group-sport endeavors. These activities can occur through family, school, work, and neighborhood associations. They interconnect to the SDOH domain of social and community context, as well as neighborhood and built environment. The social connections that occur through any of these pursuits make it possible for individuals and communities to flourish when they are found to be supportive but experience declining health when they do not exist or are toxic.[11,12] The ability for people to have exposures and experiences that promote social connectedness and belonging, or what is made possible through activities that stem from play, is a key component to thriving in life. Additionally, it supports the development of resilient mechanisms that help with coping during difficult or stressful life events. This is an important concept when considering adverse childhood experiences (ACEs) because it is understood that having access to supportive structures or people can counter the effects of ACEs.[13]

Another area that is not frequently considered in patient care is worship, or what may be referred to as spirituality or religion. It is often asked during intake processes as a way to respect cultural differences but not utilized to also note the impression it has on engaging in behaviors that are risky and unhealthy.[14] Understanding the interplay of spirituality and/or religion as part of SDOH domains that include neighborhood and built environment, social and community context, and education and literacy is another crucial component to improving outcomes for patients and communities. It has long been understood that leaders of religious entities/groups have an ability to influence their congregations in the health choices they make.[15] Support for preventive screening, vaccinations, and general health maintenance can often be heard during the announcements across the country for churchgoers. The ability for church leaders to inform and encourage health behaviors is further supported through difficulties seen during coronavirus disease 2019 (COVID-19) pandemic because it required a decrease in social interaction. The virtual options for participation in these services were implemented and are still used today to allow for continued engagement with congregants that are not able to attend physically.[16,17]

Exploring the influence of work, play, and worship within these domains on a patient's health is a difficult task overall but especially so when considering the already limited time providers have with their patients. Additionally, not being able to immediately quantify returns on investment can be seen as a barrier to hospital systems and ambulatory care settings adoption of these practices.[18] However, there are numerous resources available that can be used to advance the care of the patient to help with obtaining optimal health (**Box 1**). The key to utilization of these resources is to know that it cannot occur in a silo and that the incorporation of multidisciplinary treatment plans is a crucial part.[19–21] This article will explore the health effects of work, play, and worship as SDOH and what a primary care provider can do to impact change for their patients and communities.

WORK

Since the early 1700s when the father of Occupational Medicine, Bernadino Ramazzini, presented his seminal book cataloging toxicities and other maladies from the workplace, work has been understood to impact health. Poor work environments or bad working conditions can be associated with a multitude of health effects including

Box 1
Resources for assistance with identifying programs or organizations in other neighborhoods

General Resources:
https://nasdoh.org/resources/
https://healthleadsusa.org/resources/the-health-leads-screening-toolkit/
https://sdh-tools-review.kpwashingtonresearch.org/find-tools/submit/715

Work:

Appendix A. Relationship Between Care Model and Health Literacy Universal Precautions Toolkit
https://www.skillup.org/resource/earn-and-learn-how-to-learn-new-skills-on-the-job-and-build-your-career/

Play:
https://www.hopkinsmedicine.org/howard_county_general_hospital/services/population_health/journey_to_better_health/
https://www.cdc.gov/howrightnow/index.html

Worship:

The HOPE Questions for a Formal Spiritual Assessment in a Medical Interview
http://www.uphs.upenn.edu/pastoral/resed/diversity_points.html

cardiovascular disease,[22] mood disorders,[23] cancer,[24] and respiratory illnesses[25] among other adverse health issues. Although workplaces have oversight through the Occupational Safety and Health Administration, as well as ongoing research to inform needed changes in workplace exposures through the National Institutes of Occupational Safety and Health, the ability to protect communities and the people that are most affected requires the support of multiple aspects of health care, including the primary care clinician.[26]

An area that is often overlooked in patient care but has a role to play in each of the domains outlined by *Healthy People 2030* is work. The type of job, level of income, and the workplace environment can all contribute to the improvement or deleterious impacts of a person's health.[7] In thinking about the domains (see **Fig. 1**) that make up SDOHs, the ability to thrive in life is thought to start from the socioeconomic status of the family. Individuals that are less likely to grow up with financial stability, receive access to a quality education, live in areas that are healthy and thereby be able to access quality health care, and have a community that supports each other are understood to be more likely to not only perpetuate the same but also have worse health outcomes.[27–29] Understanding how work is influenced by each domain will further understanding of the importance of considering SDOHs in the clinic.

The domain of economic stability includes the capacity for people to afford basic needs on a consistent basis such as food, housing, and health care.[30,31] Steady employment can be the difference between being able to experience the connections from all aspects of SDOHs to include where a person lives and what type of education, as well as community programs they have access to which further supports networking, or social and community, capabilities. Although there is an understanding that economic stability is not just about having a job but also consideration of what kind of job you are doing and the potential for environmental hazards to occur, there can be pitfalls associated with steady work too. People who have experienced workplace violence, injuries, or otherwise poor working conditions may also struggle with economic stability because it relates to their personal health and ability to continue performing their role. Until livable wages and other employment programs or policies that support workers at all levels with common threats to maintaining employment such as access to child-care, educational needs, and helping with access to transportation and food, workers will continue to be impacted by this domain.

Education access and quality is directly linked to the ability for people to achieve high-paying roles and responsibilities.[29] Understanding that there are many barriers to accessing quality education, being able to draw on financial, personal, and community support provides the foundation to completing ones training, let alone the capacity to enter and complete higher levels of instruction. It is further understood that with the lack of education, whether it is due to poor quality or the inability to access it, has impacts on other SDOHs.[32] The ability for a person to meet their social and personal needs is directly linked to income production and thereby educational attainment. One study concluded that years of potential life lost was inversely associated with educational attainment.[33,34] It is due to this construct that underscores the need to identify and discuss resources that can help a patient disrupt their current situation to engage in paths that will lead to increased opportunities and suspected health. It will further support the ability for people to likely improve their lives across the other 4 domains that make up the SDOHs.

Improving a person's circumstances through economic stability and education can help with accessing necessary support systems. The ties to social and community context, neighborhood and built environment, and health access and quality are easily linked to the above domains. However, the ability to do this is the hard part. Workers need a way to advance their skills, know there is support system to help, and resources to make the changes necessary. The areas that can be championed through primary care include helping to connect the patient with the right resources including use of a social worker or other health-care team member who understands what programs may be available. Along with this, the need to adopt a health literacy model into the practice will better support the patient's understanding of what is being done, as well as outcomes from these changes.[35] What is unfortunately not possible from a primary care standpoint is the ability to change the conditions within the workplace. However, advocating with and for the patient to obtain the skills needed to better their circumstances and overall health will exclude this difficulty for the patient.

PLAY

There is a wealth of support for the need for humans to have social connections and interactions.[36] The built environment, socioeconomic status, and educational attainment of a person and their family have a notable connection to the health and mortality for that person.[32,37,38] The health effects that occur due to lack of play, or people not having the ability to socialize with others, is understood to be connected to mental health and even physical ailments. These aspects of living that relate to the proximity of healthy foods, safe spaces, health care, and safe people can all be connected to the supportive structures necessary for increasing opportunities for play.

The environment that allows for a person to grow and flourish is understood to be one that encompasses social cohesion, as well as notable family resilience.[39,40] The encouragement obtained from family members, neighbors, and others helps to shape and mold them into the adults they become. With incidents of ACEs and inefficient or nonexistent support systems, the risk of unsafe and unhealthy behaviors is amplified.[13] This is the basis for understanding the need for the domains of social and community context, as well as the neighborhood and built environment. The concept of play as a SDOH has direct and ongoing linkages to childhood. The need to protect children from the barrage of experiences that could lead to the self-harming behaviors of substance use and risky sexual interactions, as well as obesity, can occur with attention to these nonmedical aspects of health care.[41,42]

The Community Preventive Services Task Force supports the use of out-of-school programs to help improve health equity for low-income communities including those of racial and ethnic minority demographics.[42,43] Participation in these types of programs is also noted to protect children from substance use disorders because research demonstrates adolescents have a higher likelihood of use with unsupervised time. A key takeaway from this is for the possibility of primary care providers to engage in meaningful conversations related to access to these types of programs. Still noting the time constraints during clinic visits, this could also be provided in the way of literature that is available in the waiting room or posted in the clinic room or common areas. Similarly, a social worker or other resource could be used to help with ensuring this interaction occurs.

Although the above is one avenue to consider in the intersection of play as an SDOH, the consideration of older individuals and the need for a sense of community, as well as being able to live in a safe area is also vital to achieving better health.[27] The relative causes span across the built and social environment components of these living spaces to include the actual human-made structures of poverty-stricken areas that are often found to be in dilapidated conditions, as well as the lack of access to activities, places, or organizations that would be beneficial in creating the needed supportive environment.[44] Individuals suffer from depression, increased rates of cancer, lack of physical activity, and incorporation of other undesirable habits that directly affect their health. The care that is already given during clinic visits to treat these conditions are needed but if additional resources were included to support identifying ways to support healthy interactions, this would support better outcomes in the health of the individual and community. This could occur with both the use of multidisciplinary teams who know and understand the areas that the patient lives in and social prescribing.[45] Primary care providers are uniquely positioned to support their patients by providing detailed resources that will help the patient engage in helpful, community-based activities.

Ultimately, the concept of play as an SDOH is engrained in the established adage *it takes a village to raise a child*. Coupled with this is also the understanding that humans are a social species. Although this concept would be considered by some as a nonmedical concern or scope, the literature is clear about the medical impact from having to live through conditions where varying types of social interaction are necessary to thrive. It is increasingly important to ensure the incorporation of plans that include considerations around a patient's community and home-life if the expectation for a favorable outcome is to occur. Primary care providers, along with their support staff and other specialists, can and should discuss home and community situations that would limit adherence or even initiation of their treatment plan.

WORSHIP

The majority of people acknowledge participation in some form of religious or spiritual practice.[46] Literature supports that there are positive and negative impacts from participating or not participating in either religious or spiritual activities.[14] These findings support that people who do not participate in worship practices are more likely to engage in risky health behaviors, as well as have more frequent physical and mental health issues.[47] In contrast, recovery from various physical and mental health issues is thought to be improved if there are religious or spiritual practices involved.[48] It is further understood that religious practices are associated with lower odds of death when faced with health concerns.[49] Consideration of these findings implicates the need to include religious and spiritual discussions in health care as a way to improve health outcomes for a substantial subset of patients.

Contemplating the idea of religion or spirituality as a possible means to improving health care can be a subject that some may be very uncomfortable approaching. More recent inclusions in medical or health-care training include cultural sensitivity, which often times discusses religious practices for various people. With this introduction to religious or spiritual practices, the expected endgame is to ensure patients feel respected and providers have some background on things that should or should not occur with their patients.[50] Inclusion of cultural, religious, and spiritual values is written into requirements by The Joint Commission, noting the importance of respecting the wishes and needs of the patient in the provision of care. Although literature supports that this is also important because it pertains to improved health outcomes, what is likely not readily considered by health-care providers is the influence religion or spirituality has on the actual health of the patient.

Worship as an SDOH is inclusive of both religious and spiritual practices. Religion is understood to be more specific pursuit within faith-based system and includes the worship of an entity or entities, whereas spirituality is more fluid and focuses more on the values of religion but typically includes a belief in something greater than that person. The important aspect of patients that engage in spiritual or religious activities is their ability to make safer and more healthful choices.[14] It is suggested that the sense of community experienced and the social supports provided through these practices encourage these behaviors. A study completed during the COVID-19 pandemic found that the use of remote worship participation left some with unmet needs due to difficulty with accessing previously utilized social interactions.[16,17]

In consideration of the necessity noted in these social interactions, the domains most affected through SDOH are neighborhood and built environment and social and community context, along with education and literacy. Typically, worship services or activities are set in the neighborhoods that they service with the intent to increase access and provide the needed social engagement from the pulpit to the congregation. Places of worship provide a public gathering space and can be supportive with not only social interaction but also with supplying support through meals, and various types of information (ie, community involvement, health promotion, or educational programs).[51] Faith leaders are the guiding voice through these efforts and can help or hinder the progress needed to ensure protection with activities that are known to prevent morbidity and mortality from various diseases.[52] Reflecting on this paradigm indicates the importance of developing community partnerships with religious entities to understand the needs of the area being served but also to improve resources for those in need.

In the clinic, the use of cultural sensitivity with patients continues to be needed and will help to improve communication and utilization of treatment plans. However, enhancing this with additional interactions that includes discussions around religious or spiritual practices can be beneficial to further understand the potential pitfalls of a patient. It also provides the opportunity for the provider or member of the health-care team to help identify worship centers that are in line with the patient's worship practices to further support the patient's needs. This connection should not stop with simply giving literature or having a discussion with the patient but also engaging with the faith-based leaders to increase indirect access to their congregations and thereby the health messaging needed. Although it is important to consider religious and spiritual practices of patients and how to help with increasing access for them, it should not be confused with needing to engage with or offer religious or spiritual advice. Nonetheless, primary care providers can further their rapport with patients through these interactions and improved use of multidisciplinary health teams.

CLINICS CARE POINTS

- Help patients connect with the right resources including use of a social worker or other health-care team member who understands what programs may be available
- Adopt a health literacy model into the practice will better support the patient's understanding of what is being done, as well as outcomes from these changes
- Advocate with and for the patient to obtain the skills needed to better their circumstances and overall health
- Engage in meaningful conversations related to access to out-of-school programs for adolescents
- Provide literature in the waiting room or posted in the clinic room or common areas
- Provide detailed resources that will help the patient engage in helpful, community-based activities
- Discuss home and community situations that would limit adherence or even initiation of a treatment plan
- Use community partnerships to provide resources to patients that could be beneficial to their overall health (ie, listing of community organizations, churches, and activities)
- Use a multidisciplinary team to assist with providing appropriate and sensitive resources to the patient

DISCLOSURE

There are no actual or suspected conflicts of interest in relation to the provided information.

REFERENCES

1. Sable MR, Schild DR, Hipp JA. Public health and social work. In: Gehlert S, Browne T, editors. Handbook of health social work. 2nd ed. New Jersey: John Wiley and Sons; 2012. p. 64–99.
2. Buhler-Wilkerson K. Bringing care to the people: Lillian Wald's legacy to public health nursing. Am J Public Health 1993;83(12):1778–86.
3. Fee E, Garofalo ME. Florence Nightingale and the Crimean War. Am J Public Health 2010;100(9):1591, published correction appears in Am J Public Health. 2011 May;101(5):776.
4. Available at: https://www.who.int/health-topics/social-determinants-of-health#tab=tab_1. Accessed October 3, 2022.
5. Healthy People 2030, U.S. Department of Health and Human Services, Office of Disease Prevention and Health Promotion. Retrieved [October 18, 2022]. Available at: https://health.gov/healthypeople/objectives-and-data/social-determinants-health.
6. Levy BS, Wegman DH, Baron SL, et al. Chemical Hazards and Physical Hazards. In: *Occupational and Environmental Health*. 6th ed. Oxford University Press; 2011. p. 192–280.

7. Burgard SA, Lin KY. Bad Jobs, Bad Health? How Work and Working Conditions Contribute to Health Disparities. Am Behav Sci 2013;57(8). https://doi.org/10.1177/0002764213487347.
8. Hergenrather K, Zeglin R, McGuire-Kuletz M, et al. Employment as a social determinant of health: a systematic review of longitudinal studies exploring the relationship between employment status and physical health. Rehabilitation Research 2015;29(1). https://doi.org/10.1891/2168-6653.29.1.2.
9. Lynch JW, Kaplan GA. Understanding how inequality in the distribution of income affects health. J Health Psychol 1997;2(3):297–314.
10. Cheng TL, Johnson SB, Goodman E. Breaking the Intergenerational Cycle of Disadvantage: The Three Generation Approach. Pediatrics 2016;137(6). e20152467.
11. Holt-Lunstad J, Smith TB, Layton JB. Social relationships and mortality risk: a meta-analytic review. PLoS Med 2010;7(7):e1000316.
12. Meisters R, Putrik P, Westra D, et al. Is Loneliness an Undervalued Pathway between Socio-Economic Disadvantage and Health? Int J Environ Res Public Health 2021;18(19):10177.
13. McEwen C, Gregerson SF. A critical assessment of the adverse childhood experiences study at 20 years. Am J Prev Med 2019;56(6):790–4. Published:February 23, 2019.
14. Chatters LM. Religion and health: public health research and practice. Annu Rev Public Health 2000;21:335–67.
15. Anshel MH, Smith M. The role of religious leaders in promoting healthy habits in religious institutions. J Relig Health 2014;53:1046–59.
16. Kretzler B, König HH, Hajek A. Utilization of internet for religious purposes and psychosocial outcomes during the COVID-19 pandemic. Arch Gerontol Geriatr 2023;108:104900.
17. Mosavel M, Hoadley A, Akinkugbe AA, et al. Religiosity and COVID-19: Impact on Use of Remote Worship and Changes in Self-Reported Social Support. Int J Environ Res Public Health 2022;19(16):9891.
18. Parrill RE. A framework for developing, implementing, and evaluating a social determinants of health initiative. J Healthc Manag 2020;65(4):256–64.
19. Butkus R, Rapp K, Cooney TG, et al. Health and public policy committee of the american college of physicians. Envisioning a Better U.S. Health care system for all: reducing barriers to care and addressing social determinants of health. Ann Intern Med 2020;172:S50–9.
20. Thornton RL, Glover CM, Cené CW, et al. Evaluating strategies for reducing health disparities by addressing the social determinants of health. Health Aff 2016;35(8):1416–23.
21. Leibel S, Geng B, Phipatanakul W, et al. Screening social determinants of health in a multidisciplinary severe asthma clinical program. Pediatr Qual Saf 2020;5(5):e360.
22. Kivimäki M, Kawachi I. Work stress as a risk factor for cardiovascular disease. Curr Cardiol Rep 2015;17(74). https://doi.org/10.1007/s11886-015-0630-8.
23. Woo JM, Postolache TT. The impact of work environment on mood disorders and suicide: Evidence and implications. Int J Disabil Hum Dev 2008;7(2):185–200.
24. Eguchi H, Wada K, Prieto-Merino D, et al. Lung, gastric and colorectal cancer mortality by occupation and industry among working-aged men in Japan. Sci Rep 2017;7:43204.
25. Harber P, Redlich CA, Henneberger PK. Work-related lung diseases. Am J Respir Crit Care Med 2016;193(2):P3–4.

26. Buijs P, Gunnyeon B, van Weel C. Primary health care: what role for occupational health? Br J Gen Pract 2012;62(605):623–4.
27. Khullar D. Health, income, and poverty: where we are and what could help. health policy brief. Health Aff 2018. https://doi.org/10.1377/hpb20180817.901935.
28. Banaji MR, Fiske ST, Massey DS. Systemic racism: individuals and interactions, institutions and society. Cogn. Research 2021;82. https://doi.org/10.1186/s41235-021-00349-3.
29. Zajacova A, Lawrence EM. The relationship between education and health: reducing disparities through a contextual approach. Annu Rev Public Health 2018;39(1):273–89.
30. Kreuter MW, Thompson T, McQueen A, et al. Addressing social needs in health care settings: evidence, challenges, and opportunities for public health. Annu Rev Public Health 2021;42(1):329–44.
31. Andermann A, CLEAR Collaboration. Taking action on the social determinants of health in clinical practice: a framework for health professionals. CMAJ (Can Med Assoc J) 2016;188(17–18):E474–83.
32. Braveman P, Gottlieb L. The social determinants of health: it's time to consider the causes of the causes. Public Health Rep 2014;129(Suppl 2):19–31.
33. Montez JK, Hummer RA, Hayward MD. Educational attainment and adult mortality in the United States: a systematic analysis of functional form. Demography 2012;49(1):315–36.
34. Roy B, Kiefe CI, Jacobs DR, et al. Education, race/ethnicity, and causes of premature mortality among middle-aged adults in 4 US urban communities: results from CARDIA, 1985–2017. Am J Public Health 2020;110:530–6.
35. Koh HK, Brach C, Harris LM, et al. A proposed 'health literate care model' would constitute a systems approach to improving patients' engagement in care. Health Aff 2013;32(2):357–67.
36. Umberson D, Montez JK. Social relationships and health: a flashpoint for health policy. J Health Soc Behav 2010;51(Suppl):S54–66.
37. McMaughan DJ, Oloruntoba O, Smith ML. Socioeconomic Status and Access to Healthcare: Interrelated Drivers for Healthy Aging. Front Public Health 2020; 8:231.
38. Hankey S, Marshall JD, Brauer M. Health impacts of the built environment: within-urban variability in physical inactivity, air pollution, and ischemic heart disease mortality. Environ Health Perspect 2012;120:2.
39. Jennings V, Bamkole O. The relationship between social cohesion and urban green space: an avenue for health promotion. Int J Environ Res Public Health 2019;16(3):452.
40. Barnhart S, Bode M, Gearhart MC, et al. Supportive neighborhoods, family resilience and flourishing in childhood and adolescence. Children 2022;9(4):495.
41. Atashbahar O, Sari AA, Takian A, et al. The impact of social determinants of health on early childhood development: a qualitative context analysis in Iran. BMC Public Health 2022;22(1):1149. Published 2022 Jun 8.
42. Lee KT, Vandell DL. Out-of-School Time and Adolescent Substance Use. J Adolesc Health 2015;57(5):523–9.
43. Available at: https://www.thecommunityguide.org/findings/social-determinants-health-out-school-time-academic-programs-general.html. Accessed: January 7, 2023.
44. Hood E. Dwelling disparities: how poor housing leads to poor health. Environ Health Perspect 2005;113(5):A310–7.

45. Bild E, Pachana NA. Social prescribing: a narrative review of how community engagement can improve wellbeing in later life. J Community Appl Soc Psychol 2022;32(6):1148–215.
46. Oxhandler HK, Polson EC, Achenbaum WA. The religiosity and spiritual beliefs and practices of clinical social workers: a national survey. Soc Work 2018; 63(1):47–56.
47. George LK, Larsons DB, Koeing HG, et al. Spirituality and health: what we know, what we need to know. J Soc Clin Psychol 2000;19(1):102. Psychology Module pg.
48. Mueller PS, Plevak DJ, Rummans TA. Religious involvement, spirituality, and medicine: implications for clinical practice. Mayo Clin Proc 2001;76:1225–35.
49. McCullough ME, Hoyt WT, Larson DB, et al. Religious involvement and mortality: a meta-analytic review. Health Psychol 2000;19(3):211–22.
50. Swihart DL, Yarrarapu SNS, Martin RL. Cultural Religious Competence In Clinical Practice. [Updated 2022 Nov 14]. In: StatPearls [Internet]. Treasure Island (FL): StatPearls Publishing; 2023 Jan-. Available at: https://www.ncbi.nlm.nih.gov/books/NBK493216/. Accessed: October 12, 2022.
51. Powell TW, West KR, Turner CE. Size matters: addressing social determinants of health through black churches. J Racial Ethn Health Disparities 2021;8(1): 237–44.
52. Heward-Mills NL, Atuhaire C, Spoors C, et al. The role of faith leaders in influencing health behaviour: a qualitative exploration on the views of Black African Christians in Leeds, United Kingdom. Pan Afr Med J 2018;30:199.

Food and Nutrition Security as Social Determinants of Health: Fostering Collective Impact to Build Equity

Duncan Y. Amegbletor, PhD[a], Danny Goldberg, MA[b], Derek A. Pope, PhD[a], Bryan W. Heckman, PhD[a,c,*]

KEYWORDS

• Food insecurity • Urban agriculture • Community engagement • Obesity • SDoH

KEY POINTS

- The existence of food deserts in America is an injustice that we have not been able to correct despite decades of effort.
- There is a parallel obesity crisis directly caused by the standard American diet.
- A new generation of local, bottom-up solutions can correct the dual crises of obesity and food insecurity that are the direct result of policy decisions and infrastructure.

PRIMARY CARE PROVIDERS CAN SHAPE POPULATION HEALTH

Poor diet is responsible for one of the every five deaths worldwide, and represents a significant risk factor for a range of chronic medical conditions.[1] Approaches to address the consumption of unhealthy foods or food deprivation and improve nutrition are increasingly being integrated into healthcare systems for the prevention, management, and treatment of chronic conditions.[2,3] Promising evidence indicates positive impacts of food and nutrition interventions for patient-provider relationship, patient satisfaction, healthcare costs, and health outcomes. However, substantial opportunities remain to optimize measurement, data integrations, effectiveness across diverse patient characteristics, scalability, reach, and sustainable implementation as a routine component of evidence-based care.[4,5]

Primary care providers (PCPs) can accelerate achieving transformative improvements to patient-centered care and health outcomes, particularly within communities

[a] Department of Psychiatry & Behavioral Sciences, Meharry Medical College, 1005 Dr. D.B. Todd, Jr. Boulevard, Nashville, TN 37208, USA; [b] Grow2Learn Cooperative, 445 Kemper Drive, North, Madison, TN 37115, USA; [c] Division of Public Health, School of Graduate Studies and Research, Meharry Medical College, 1005 Dr. D.B. Todd, Jr. Boulevard, Nashville, TN 37208, USA
* Corresponding author.
E-mail address: bheckman@mmc.edu

Prim Care Clin Office Pract 50 (2023) 633–644
https://doi.org/10.1016/j.pop.2023.05.006
primarycare.theclinics.com

where healthy foods are scarce or difficult to obtain.[6] The United States Department of Agriculture (USDA) defines the ability to access enough food for healthy life is termed *food security.*[7] *Low food security* reflects reduced quality, variety, or desirability, but negligible change in the amount of food consumption. *Very low food security* is characterized as multiple indications of disrupted eating patterns and reduced food intake. Interactive visualizations on the USDA website[7] indicate 10.2% of Americans live with food insecurity and 3.8% live with very low food security, and allow viewers to see trends over time and examine potential risk factors. Food security is a necessary, but not sufficient, driver for *nutrition security*, which further requires that the foods/beverages promote well-being, prevent disease, and, if needed, treat disease.[8,9] There is a strong body of evidence demonstrating an array of negative health consequences for those living with food/nutrition insecurity.[10,11] Disparities are most evident in communities where poverty rates are high (>20%), single-mother households, inner city or rural areas, and communities of color.[12–15] PCP-led food/nutrition interventions represent pathways for the delivery of high impact solutions to reduce these preventable causes of death, lower quality of life, multiple comorbidities, healthcare costs, and health disparities.[16]

The importance and urgency of addressing the food and nutrition-related health crisis in the U.S. prompted the White House Conference on Food, Nutrition, and Health in September 2022,[17] along with a series of listening and planning sessions across diverse stakeholders. Those with lived experience, healthcare providers, policy decision makers, researchers, and others from multiple sectors (government, private, academia, community-based organizations) contributed to a National Strategic Plan to end hunger and increase healthy eating and physical activity by 2030.

This article aims to: (1) document the impacts of food/nutrition insecurity on health outcomes; (2) examine factors that modulate food/nutrition security; (3) delineate opportunities for PCP impact; and (4) highlight innovative and promising multi-level approaches to the benefits of community health activism focused on SDoH.

FOOD & NUTRITION SECURITY AND HEALTH OUTCOMES

The significance of food is often overlooked. Food is a primary reinforcer that influences behavior across every animal on the planet, and is oftentimes a critical aspect of individual decision-making, sustained behavior, cultural norms, and historical events. We all are biologically driven to work in some manner to get food, and food consumption can strengthen the likelihood of doing the same work again. Unfortunately, underserved communities are required to "work" harder to obtain healthy foods, and this additional work may increase the reinforcement value, purchasing, and consumption of less nutritious but more easily accessible foods.

Location of residency can greatly impact food and nutrition security. *Food deserts*, as defined by the USDA, are areas with limited access to a variety of healthy and affordable food.[14,18,19] due to factors such as a long distance (>1 mile in urban areas; >10 miles in rural areas) from the closest large grocery store.[14] Oftentimes, these areas are also considered *food swamps* due to greater access, via higher density of small convenience stores, to unhealthy, calorie-dense, and inexpensive junk food and high sugar foods.[20] These environmental contexts represent social determinants of health. Moreover, the effects of these conditions produce a disproportional burden of diet-related chronic diseases observed across underserved populations, such as racial and ethnic minorities, low-income, and rural and remote populations including Tribal communities and insular areas.[15,19,21]

Consider a household that does not own a vehicle and resides in an area saturated with convenience stores and devoid of places to buy nutritious foods. These family members must expend more time and effort to obtain nutrient-rich foods relative to households with closer proximity to healthy foods. Even when there is high interest and need for healthy foods, lack of access to resources (eg, money, time, childcare needs) that may be necessary to make a shopping trip add to the burden caused by transportation. After factoring in the other SDoHs commonly experienced by households in food limited areas (eg, poverty) may further limit capacity for meeting additional "work" demands, it becomes easier to understand rationale for decision-making sustained behaviors that are unhealthy and undermine health outcomes.

The U.S. population has a rising prevalence of diet-related chronic conditions such as type 2 diabetes, obesity, hypertension, and certain cancers. These largely preventable consequences disproportionately impact historically underserved communities. Obesity leads to a higher risk for poor health outcomes such as hypertension, diabetes, high cholesterol, heart disease, and stroke.[22] Ultimately, being overweight or obese is associated with a higher risk of mortality. A large meta-analysis of over ten million participants across four continents and 239 studies found strong correlations between body mass index (BMI) and overall mortality,[23] with strongest associations observed among those considered overweight (>25 BMI).

Obesity has associations with several types of cancers due to the hormonal and inflammatory changes associated with the disease. These obesity-related cancers (eg, breast, colon, pancreatic, ovarian, thyroid) make up 40% of all diagnosed cancers and disproportionately affect women.[22] Being overweight or obese has negative effects on the cardiovascular system, although these effects can be partially mitigated by regular exercise.[24] Obesity is associated with changes to cardiac tissue culminating in impaired function and increased atrial and ventricular mass.[25] Pulmonary function is also affected by obesity[26] via increased airway pressure and chronic inflammation leading to increased risk of obstructive sleep apnea, obesity-hypoventilation syndrome, and asthma.[25] Similarly, the chronic inflammation in obese individuals has been identified as a risk factor for Alzheimer's disease.[27–29]

Furthermore, diet can have deleterious effects on emotional and psychological outcomes. Adults living with food/nutrition insecurity have been found at greater risk for depression/anxiety and lower quality of life.[30]Food insecurity experienced during childhood may contribute to both acute and long-term mental health consequences. Reduced academic performance, deficits in impulse control, and exacerbated symptoms of attention-deficit hyperactivity disorder have been associated with nutrition deficits, likely due to disrupting neurocognitive develpment.[31,32] During adulthood, there may be increased risk for depression, interpersonal violence, suicidal ideation, and substance use disorder[33] The Mediterranean diet (as well as the "epigenetic diet") has been shown to be protective for mental disorders.[34]

RISK FACTORS AND PROTECTIVE BUFFERS: LONG-STANDING DISCRIMINATION

Disparities in food/nutrition security have been generated and perpetuated by structural racism embedded within policies and practices. Social, economic, and legal discrimination institutionalized by Black codes and Jim Crow laws continue to harm Black communities. For instance, the Southeastern U.S. (HHS Region IV) has the highest levels of food insecurity, as well as many other economic and health disparities. *Food apartheid* was coined to be distinct from food/nutrition by integrating intentional discrimination that has produced relevant environmental contexts (eg, food desert/swamp), alongside many other contributors to food insecurity: residential segregation, deepened poverty, supermarket relocation, and ignorance among white populations of the foodways of Black, Brown, and Indigenous communities. Examples include limited urban farming due to zoning policies, economic and social impacts caused by historic redlining, or limited access to farm capital based on federal subsidy and loan programs. Higher food insecurity is found in neighborhoods in areas which were never industrialized or were de-industrialized.[21] U.S. food insecurity is partially a consequence of regional and local infrastructural related to the economics of food distribution, and not an issue of the nation lacking the food necessary to feed all residents. Economic pressures lead to food distributors concentrating stores in high-wealth neighborhoods where selling food will be more profitable, resulting in food deserts/swamps.

Financial barriers at multiple levels of analysis impede equitable food/nutrition security. Households that are food secure spend nearly 20% more on food compared to food-insecure households, even after considering household size, composition, and federal assistance programs. Providing subsidized or free healthy food can reduce obesogenic diets, as well as taxation/prices increases for unhealthy foods. Interventions that address access to quality food only can overcome geographical barriers, such as high-quality food assistance.[19] Low-income households that received housing vouchers for relocation to lower-poverty areas had lower rates of extreme obesity and diabetes over a 10-year follow-up, although household income had not increased compared to their counterparts.[35] There is an urgent need to overcome the cycle of diet-related disparities produced from social injustice and SDoH, such as the 10-fold higher transgenerational wealth observed in white versus black families that has persisted for over 70 years.

Inclusive food governance is another major issue undermining food/nutrition security.[36] U.S. National Strategic Plan represents an important collective impact initiative that promotes more inclusive approaches. Five pillars guide calls to action and over eight-billion-dollar federal budget were dedicated to eliminating diet-related diseases.

1. *Improving food access and affordability*, including by advancing economic security; increasing access to free and nourishing school meals; providing Summer Electronic Benefits Transfer (EBT) benefits to more children; and expanding Supplemental Nutrition Assistance Program (SNAP) eligibility to more underserved populations.
2. *Integrating nutrition and health*, including by working with Congress to pilot coverage of medically tailored meals in Medicare; testing Medicaid coverage of nutrition education and other nutrition supports using Medicaid section 1115 demonstration projects; and expanding Medicaid and Medicare beneficiaries' access to nutrition and obesity counseling.
3. *Empowering all consumers* to make and have access to healthy choices, including by proposing to develop a front-of-package labeling scheme for food packages; proposing to update the nutrition criteria for the "healthy" claim on food packages; expanding incentives for fruits and vegetables in SNAP; facilitating sodium reduction in the food supply by issuing longer-term, voluntary sodium targets for industry; and assessing additional steps to reduce added sugar consumption, including potential voluntary targets.
4. *Supporting physical activity* for all, including by expanding the U.S. Department of Health and Human Services' Centers for Disease Control and Prevention's (CDC) State Physical Activity and Nutrition Program to all states and territories; investing in efforts to connect people to parks and other outdoor spaces; and funding regular updates to and promotion of the Physical Activity Guidelines for Americans.

5. *Enhancing nutrition and food security research*, including by bolstering funding to improve metrics, data collection, and research to inform nutrition and food security policy, particularly on issues of equity and access; and implementing a vision for advancing nutrition science.

PRIMARY CARE PROVIDER-LED OPPORTUNITIES TO ACCELERATE FOOD/NUTRITION SECURITY

PCPs and associated clinic personnel have unique opportunities to enhance food/nutrition security. Patients speak to these healthcare providers about their health most frequently and provide care for extended durations. Key roles and major areas of leadership and involvement include the harmonization of assessment/data collection through the use of validated screening tools[18,37] (Food Insecurity-hl7.org; SDOH & Practice Improvement) interoperability and outcome measurement standards; expansion of sites of care to increase reach and potential utilization; scale and disseminate interventions, including partnerships with community-based organizations. Standardization will allow all stakeholders to better communicate and address food/nutrition insecurity. Primary care clinics can serve as access points to food/nutrition interventions directly or as a pipeline to connect patients to the organizations/networks that provide them.[4,38] Benefits to health outcomes have been observed after screening, intervening, or referring were added to PCP workflows designed to address SDoH.[39] This approach results in more personalized treatment plans and better meets unique patient needs and priorities, expanding beyond one-size-fits-all approaches. A review of approximately 200 studies across four chronic conditions found that illness and treatment burden combined with general demands and resources (eg, SDoH) predicts treatment engagement and health outcomes through perceived treatment fatigue. Personalized and patient-centered care that better meet patients' priorities and needs (eg, SDoH) may mitigate fatigue and increase sustained engagement and health outcomes.[40]

PCPs should have the expertise to ask and counsel patients about food insecurity, and the capacity to refer and link patients to food assistance resources.[41] Partnerships with community-based organizations can address potential barriers for clinic implementation (time, training, and access to resources). For example, health systems and neighborhood food pantries, farmers markets, and/or community gardens have enhanced patient care through produce prescription programs, nutrition education, and enrollment in federal assistance.

Knowledge of federal assistance programs and integrating referrals as part of a typical PCP visit can alleviate patient' financial barriers. The three largest federal nutrition assistance programs are Supplemental Nutrition Assistance Program (SNAP), Supplemental Nutrition Program for Women, Infants, and Children (WIC), and the National School Lunch Program. At least one of these programs is used each month by nearly 60% of food-insecure households. Referrals through primary care clinics as part of SDoH screening procedures have become more commonplace. However, it is important providers are aware of SNAP limitations,[10,42] such as: strict means testing, funding that is inflexible in times of extreme need, difficulty of SNAP benefits alone in eliminating food insecurity. Ideally, information about complementary options can be shared, most of which will include local community-based organizations.

Food is medicine interventions are designed to improve health outcomes specifically and have been associated with better chronic disease management and lower hospital admissions.[4,43] Medically-tailored meal, grocery (food pharmacies), and produce prescriptions are promising approaches, which may improve the ability to adhere to dietary recommendations by overcoming access and affordability barriers.[16,44] Benefits associated with this approach can be calculated via online tools[45] (https://www.dietid.com/roi-calculator) to provide objective metrics to monitor impact and further promote adoption or modifications. Training for providers can ensure adequate competencies, enhance the dissemination of shared resources, and standardize the delivery of SDoH-driven care (https://lifestylemedicine.org/). Promoting behavior change in other unhealthy behaviors can also support food security. For example, smoking cessation has been linked with lower food insecurity risk, likely due to reduced spending on cigarettes that can help alleviate financial barriers to healthy food purchases. Additionally, lifestyle changes consistent with longevity and wellbeing can be supported, such as stress management, healthy sleep, community building, activity, and sense of purpose (Live Better, Longer - Blue Zones).

PCPs can further shape population health through research collaborations that develop, evaluate, disseminate, and implement novel approaches. Later in discussion, we describe promising approaches that will benefit from PCP leadership and role as trusted messengers to raise awareness within communities regarding participation in ongoing research trials and community health activism efforts. Finally, PCPs can advocate for policies that support food/nutrition security and maintain workplace wellness programs to support staff and self-care.

Case Study Example

A 30-year-old single mother of two brings her two children in for routine immunizations. During the visit, she is screened for food insecurity as part of routine screening for SDoH as recommended by the AAP. The screening reveals the mother always feels anxious that her food supply will run out before her next paycheck. She further reveals that sometimes she is unable to make it to the grocery store – and she says she is just too tired to get off the bus – go to the store – then get back on the bus to travel the last 3 miles home. As a result, she often just orders pizza instead. The PCP, knowing that the new 2021 CMS billing guidelines allow for time-based billing, spends 30 minutes counseling about nutrition and food insecurity, At the end, the PCP provides a list of community-based resources including Second Harvest Food Bank, Nashville General Hospital's Food Pharmacy Program and Grow2Learn Community Co-op. The PCPs office has a "close the loop" system in place and will follow up at the next visit to see if the community referral was accepted.

PROMISING NEXT-GENERATION SOLUTIONS

Technology-based tools that complement standard care are emerging rapidly and may enhance the efficiency, effectiveness, and reach of evidence-based care. Smartphone ownership has jumped from 35% in 2011 to 85% in 2021 and may help mitigate the digital divide. Minority populations rely more on smartphone technology as a primary source for healthcare information due to disparities across other technologies. Empirically supported treatments through smartphone apps, after validated through rigorous trials, may offer the unprecedented capacity to automate and integrate data collection, support decision support tools, deliver treatment in real-time, and meet the dynamic needs of patients. PCPs can capitalize on the high reach this market affords and guide consumers to approaches that work, especially since this may increase access to treatment for those who may be unable or unwilling to seek it in person (eg, cost, distance, stigma).

The next generation of food assistance policy needs to facilitate both *access* and *affordability* of nutrient-rich food. Solutions will best meet community needs through approaches that integrate community input and are tailored to the infrastructure and material conditions of the regions/neighborhoods in question. Bringing together leaders from diverse perspectives offers the opportunity to shed light on overlooked and practical solutions with high-impact implications for restoring trust, advancing care, and amplifying the voice of underserved communities. These approaches are often driven by "bottom-up" needs rather than "top-down" decrees. The phrase "nothing about us, without us" is a recommended guiding principle. Those with lived experience are typically left out of policy decisions despite being the ones that face associated consequences. Ameliorating the effects of America's food governance must engage community members and involve more diverse stakeholders provided a seat at the table. Tools and opportunities to exert control over the production and distribution of their own food is a promising method to empower communities and overcome long-standing discrimination. Widespread local food production and distribution, especially in neighborhoods without legitimate grocery stores, overcomes barriers of affordability, access, transportation, and infrastructure. Potential to increase the sustainability of funding and scalability of the initiatives, by shifting from grant-based to cooperative investments based on mutually beneficial arrangements with long-term vision and an equity lens at the heart of the partnership. Just as the infrastructure for growing and distributing food benefits from locality, resilience and investment in this infrastructure is also strengthened by local partnerships and collaboration.

Existing models that incentivize business leaders to invest in co-operative initiatives may have potential utility to support food/nutrition security. For example, carbon offset credits trade on the measurable reduction of greenhouse gasses,[46] by directing funds to conservation and sustainable development efforts and reducing industry climate emissions. We are exploring potential parallels that can be supported via security offsets by reducing unhealthy food access and/or increasing healthy food access and reduce disparities, or potential for equity credits to compensate for other SDoH produces by various industries. For example, policies could be enacted to require organizations responsible for SDoH that produce or maintain food/nutrition insecurity to redirect funds (eg, social impact investments or offset credits) and promote population health. May offer avenue for sustainable funds for social profit entities, de-incentive pro-SDoH company behaviors, and foster investor incentives through market competition that applies return on investment strategies to non-profit sector operations.[47,48] We are optimistic this paradigm shift may produce transformative impact by promulgating scalable and sustainable systems level change to increase healthy behavior and ameliorate SDoHs (stabilize housing, poverty), discrimination, trauma, and disparities.[46] Rigorous evaluations designed and led by cross-sector coalitions are underway to test these hypotheses.

Healing-centered design approaches shift conceptualizations from personal decrements to community solutions and use gain-versus loss-framed language to promote community empowerment and collective solutions. For example, "determinants of food *insecurity* and *patient* outcomes are difficult to change because they are caused by *deeply rooted, complex* interactions, across *multiple levels of analysis" can be reframed to* "the breadth of contributors to food *security* represents many *pathways to produce positive outcomes* (trust, quality, and quantity of care, engagement, outcomes, and cost savings) that can *benefit population health*." Community-level SDoH stabilization is supported by improving local access to healthy food and neighborhood-driven interventions and governance.[49] Culture and restoration of identity are central elements used to build solid sense of meaning, self-perception, purpose, and belonging.[50] Food co-ops organize people to discover where food products come from and how food can facilitate connectedness and cultures of health. Cohesiveness within communities has been shown to mitigate food insecurity, likely a result of shared resource allocation (eg, transportation).[21] Food co-ops use immersive education, training, and employment programs to make agricultural experiences accessible for all.

The COVID-19 pandemic demonstrated the fragility of global supply chains. Local food infrastructure may be more likely to keep communities fed in times of crisis, rather than top-down responses that may be delayed or nonresponsive to community needs.[51–53] To change the status quo, we encourage interactive approaches to both learn and teach (mentee-mentor; peer-based) integrative food systems, historical and cultural relevance, and collective capacity for growing, preparation, cooking, eating, entrepreneurship and celebrating the change we wish to see: innovative regenerative and resilient community-led economic models that build community resilience and expands instead of extracting resources and dissolving neighborhoods.

Food is our common ground, a universal experience.

—James Beard

DISCUSSION

A health equity lens is essential when examining food and nutrition security. People who experience food insecurity have higher risk for poor nutrition[54] and diet-related conditions,[55] including obesity, diabetes, hypertension, coronary disease, stroke, and cancer. These risks are founded in long-standing SDoH,[56] https://www.ncbi.nlm.nih.gov/books/NBK425848/, such as structural racism and other structural inequities based on income, education, age, sex, place of residence, and national geography.

We provide an overview of evidence that access is necessary but not sufficient to eliminate longstanding food apartheid (food insecurity) that disproportionately harms racial and ethnic minorities and other underserved communities. Disrupting the cyclical status quo caused by long-standing discrimination, SDoHs, and health disparities to accelerate transformative impact will require multi-level collective impact approaches, inclusive of diverse stakeholders/perspectives across multiple sectors. Successful food/nutrition security solutions will have transdiagnostic implications for SDoHs broadly and other domains/conditions.

Racial and ethnic minorities will most benefit from effective solutions to promote greater food & nutrition security necessary to reduce diet-related chronic conditions, complex comorbidities, and long-standing health disparities. Specific recommendations from current best practices and resources to support ongoing training and resource sharing provide actional next steps and tools for objective measurement and tools to support population health. Innovative and promising future directions suggest an optimistic opportunity for PCPs and communities served to accelerate the elimination of disparities and broad variety of options to optimize outcomes for all. The benefits of community health activism approaches that engage and empower communities through local health programs can support cohesiveness, resource sharing, and sustainable solutions (eg, case studies, resources, videos, and more). Cross-sectoral, multi-level, approaches that are guided by community members are critical for sustainable solutions.

CLINICS CARE POINTS

- Primary care clinics offer high reach contexts to identify, assess, and intervene upon food/nutrition security needs.

- Supplemental Nutrition Assistance Program (SNAP) referrals are necessary but not sufficient. SNAP recipients still struggle with the reality of living in a food desert.
- Think of dietary choice as an environmentally dependent behavior. *Access to food* and *affordability of food* are both considerations when addressing an individual's case.
- Making connections with local community organizations can provide new sources of access for patients and overcome barriers caused by policy and infrastructure.
- Healthcare professionals and organizations can bolster the work being done by community organizations by entering multistakeholder partnerships that enhance the strength of communities and health equity.

FUNDING

This work was supported by the National Institutes of Health (K23DA041616, P50MD017347, P30AI110527) and the United States Economic Development Administration (ED22ATL3030041).

ACKNOWLEDGMENTS

The authors gratefully acknowledge Andrée LeQuire and Jafee Judah of the Grow2Learn Cooperative and Clinton Hopkins of Meharry Medical College for their support, advice, and encouragement in the development of this article.

REFERENCES

1. Murray CJL. The Global Burden of Disease Study at 30 years. Nat Med 2022; 28(10):2019–26.
2. Gu N, Kulich J, Deutsch H, Laczkowski T. Advancing health equity: Practical solutions to address variations in care. 2022. Available at: https://www.zs.com/insights/advancing-health-equity-solutions-to-address-variations-in-care. Accessed March 21, 2023.
3. ACLM Recommendations to White House Conference on Hunger, Nutrition and Health American College of Lifestyle Medicine.
4. Downer S, Berkowitz SA, Harlan TS, et al. Food is medicine: actions to integrate food and nutrition into healthcare. BMJ 2020;369:m2482.
5. Nguyen CJ, Gold R, Mohammed A, et al. Food insecurity screening in primary care: Patterns during the COVID-19 pandemic by encounter modality. Am J Prev Med 2023. https://doi.org/10.1016/j.amepre.2023.03.014.
6. Shi L. The impact of primary care: a focused review. Scientifica 2012;2012: 432892.
7. Coleman-Jensen A, Rabbitt M, Gregory C, Singh A. Household Food Security in the United States in 2021. 2022. Economic Research Service Report. Available at: https://www.ers.usda.gov/webdocs/publications/104656/err-309.pdf?v=8824.5. Accessed February 21, 2023.
8. Mozaffarian D. Measuring And Addressing Nutrition Security To Achieve Health And Health Equity. March 30, 2023.
9. Thorndike AN, Gardner CD, Kendrick KB, et al. Strengthening US food policies and programs to promote equity in nutrition security: a policy statement from the American Heart Association. Circulation 2022;145(24):e1077–93.
10. Banks AR, Bell BA, Ngendahimana D, et al. Identification of factors related to food insecurity and the implications for social determinants of health screenings. BMC Publ Health 2021;21(1):1410.

11. Lopes SO, Abrantes LCS, Azevedo FM, et al. Food Insecurity and Micronutrient Deficiency in Adults: A Systematic Review and Meta-Analysis. Nutrients 2023; 15(5):1074.
12. Beula Devamalar P, Thulasi Bai V, Srivatsa S. Design and architecture of real time web-centric telehealth diabetes diagnosis expert system. Int J Med Eng Inf 2009; 1(3):307–17.
13. Coleman-Jensen A, Nord M, Andrews M, et al. Food security in the United States in 2019. Washington, DC: US Department of Agriculture; 2019.
14. Dutko P, Ver Ploeg M, Farrigan T. Characteristics and influential factors of food deserts. 2012.
15. Elsheikh E, Barhoum N. Structural racialization and food insecurity in the United States. A Report to the UN Human Rights Committee on the International Covenant on Civil and Political Rights. 2013;20:20-26.
16. Donohue JA, Severson T, Martin LP. The food pharmacy: Theory, implementation, and opportunities. Am J Prev Cardiol 2021;5:100145.
17. House W. Biden-Harris administration national strategy on hunger, nutrition, and health. Published September 2022.
18. Lousberg C, Behal S. Food Insecurity. Gravity Project. Updated March 23, 2023. Available at: https://confluence.hl7.org/pages/viewpage.action?pageId=91994432#FoodInsecurity-Terminology,DefinitionsandResources. Accessed April 23, 2023.
19. Beverly MD. (2022) Three Essays on Food Insecurity and Economics (Doctoral dissertation, Virginia Tech).
20. Cooksey-Stowers K, Schwartz MB, Brownell KD. Food swamps predict obesity rates better than food deserts in the United States. Int J Environ Res Publ Health 2017;14(11):1366.
21. Bowen S, Elliott S, Hardison-Moody A. The structural roots of food insecurity: How racism is a fundamental cause of food insecurity. Sociology Compass 2021;15(7): e12846.
22. Cancer and Obesity. Available at: https://www.cdc.gov/vitalsigns/obesity-cancer/index.html. Accessed December 23, 3022.
23. Di Angelantonio E, Bhupathiraju SN, Wormser D, et al. Body-mass index and all-cause mortality: individual-participant-data meta-analysis of 239 prospective studies in four continents. Lancet 2016;388(10046):776–86.
24. Shaw KA, Gennat HC, O'Rourke P, Del Mar C. Exercise for overweight or obesity Cochrane database of systematic reviews. 2006;4.
25. Abdelaal M, le Roux CW, Docherty NG. Morbidity and mortality associated with obesity. Ann Transl Med 2017;5(7).
26. Koenig SM. Pulmonary Complications of Obesity. Am J Med Sci 2001;321(4): 249–79.
27. Alford S, Patel D, Perakakis N, et al. Obesity as a risk factor for Alzheimer's disease: weighing the evidence. Obes Rev 2018;19(2):269–80.
28. Pugazhenthi S, Qin L, Reddy PH. Common neurodegenerative pathways in obesity, diabetes, and Alzheimer's disease. Biochim Biophys Acta Mol Basis Dis 2017;1863(5):1037–45.
29. Profenno LA, Porsteinsson AP, Faraone SV. Meta-Analysis of Alzheimer's Disease Risk with Obesity, Diabetes, and Related Disorders. Biol Psychiatr 2010;67(6): 505–12.
30. Consequences of Obesity. 2019. Obesity Basics.
31. Melchior M, Chastang J-F, Falissard B, et al. Food insecurity and children's mental health: a prospective birth cohort study. PLoS One 2012;7(12):e52615.

32. Shankar P, Chung R, Frank DA. Association of food insecurity with children's behavioral, emotional, and academic outcomes: a systematic review. J Dev Behav Pediatr 2017;38(2):135–50.
33. McIntyre L, Williams JVA, Lavorato DH, et al. Depression and suicide ideation in late adolescence and early adulthood are an outcome of child hunger. J Affect Disord 2013;150(1):123–9.
34. Owen L, Corfe B. The role of diet and nutrition on mental health and wellbeing. Proc Nutr Soc 2017;76(4):425–6.
35. Ludwig J, Sanbonmatsu L, Gennetian L, et al. Neighborhoods, Obesity, and Diabetes — A Randomized Social Experiment. N Engl J Med 2011;365(16):1509–19.
36. Marsden T, Hebinck P, Mathijs E. Re-building food systems: embedding assemblages, infrastructures and reflexive governance for food systems transformations in Europe. Food Secur 2018;1301–9.
37. SDOH & Practice Improvement. Agency for Healthcare Research and Quality. Updated June 2021. Available at: https://www.ahrq.gov/sdoh/practice-improvement.html. Accessed April 12, 2023.
38. Brennan L, Evans M, Michaeli G, et al. Completion of Social Drivers of Health Screenings in Pediatric Practices Participating in a Quality Improvement Initiative. J Dev Behav Pediatr 2022;43(8):472–9.
39. Lundeen EA, Siegel KR, Calhoun H, et al. Peer reviewed: clinical-community partnerships to identify patients with food insecurity and address food needs. Prev Chronic Dis 2017;14.
40. Heckman BW, Mathew AR, Carpenter MJ. Treatment burden and treatment fatigue as barriers to health. Current opinion in psychology 2015;5:31–6.
41. Taher S, Persell SD, Kandula NR. Six recommendations for accelerating uptake of national food security screening in primary care settings. J Gen Intern Med 2022;1–3.
42. Serchen J, Atiq O, Hilden D. Strengthening Food and Nutrition Security to Promote Public Health in the United States: A Position Paper From the American College of Physicians. Ann Intern Med 2022;175(8):1170–1.
43. Berkowitz SA, Terranova J, Randall L, et al. Association between receipt of a medically tailored meal program and health care use. JAMA Intern Med 2019; 179(6):786–93.
44. Berkowitz SA, Shahid NN, Terranova J, et al. "I was able to eat what I am supposed to eat"–patient reflections on a medically-tailored meal intervention: a qualitative analysis. BMC Endocr Disord 2020;20:1–11.
45. Katz DL, Govani R, Anderson K, et al. The Financial Case for Food as Medicine: Introduction of a ROI Calculator. Am J Health Promot 2022;36(5):768–71.
46. Pomeroy R. Radio Davos. September. Available at: https://www.weforum.org/agenda/2022/09/carbon-offsets-radio-davos/. Accessed January 14, 2023.
47. Fraser A, Tan S, Lagarde M, et al. Narratives of Promise, Narratives of Caution: A Review of the Literature on Social Impact Bonds. Soc Pol Adm 2018;52(1):4–28.
48. Warner ME. Private finance for public goods: social impact bonds. Journal of Economic Policy Reform 2013;16(4):303–19.
49. Purcell M. The deep-down delight of democracy. Malden, MA: Wiley-Blackwell; 2013.
50. Ginwright S. The Future of Healing: Shifting From Trauma Informed Care to Healing-centered Engagement. Shawn Ginwright - Medium blog. May 31, 2018. Available at: https://ginwright.medium.com/the-future-of-healing-shifting-from-trauma-informed-care-to-healing-centered-engagement-634f557ce69c. Accessed February 8, 2023.

51. Schismenos S, Smith AA, Stevens GJ, et al. Failure to lead on COVID-19: what went wrong with the United States? International Journal of Public Leadership 2021;17(1):39–53.
52. Mener AS. Disaster response in the United States of America: An analysis of the bureaucratic and political history of a failing system. CUREJ-College Undergraduate Research Electronic Journal 2007;63.
53. Kim DKD, Kreps GL. An Analysis of Government Communication in the United States During the COVID-19 Pandemic: Recommendations for Effective Government Health Risk Communication. World Med Health Pol 2020;12(4):398–412.
54. Zhang FF, Liu J, Rehm CD, et al. Trends and Disparities in Diet Quality Among US Adults by Supplemental Nutrition Assistance Program Participation Status. JAMA Netw Open 2018;1(2):e180237.
55. Centers for Disease Control and Prevetion. Food and Nutrition Insecurity and Diabetes: Understanding the Connection. Available at: https://www.cdc.gov/diabetes/library/features/diabetes-and-food-insecurity.htm. Accessed April 28, 2023.
56. National Academies of Sciences, Engineering, and Medicine; Health and Medicine Division; Board on Population Health and Public Health Practice; Committee on Community-Based Solutions to Promote Health Equity in the United States; Baciu A, Negussie Y, Geller A, et al., editors. Communities in Action: Pathways to Health Equity. Washington (DC): National Academies Press (US); 2017. Available at: https://www.ncbi.nlm.nih.gov/books/NBK425848/. doi:10.17226/24624. Accessed April 28, 2023.

Climate Change

The Ultimate Determinant of Health

Carol Ziegler, DNP, APRN, NP-C, APHN-BC*, James Muchira, PhD, RN

KEYWORDS

- Climate change • Climate justice • Social determinants of health
- Commercial determinants of health • Carbon footprint • Allostatic load

KEY POINTS

- Climate change is the greatest threat to human health, and it influences the 5 domains of social determinants of health (SDoH).
- It disproportionately affects low-income communities of color who have contributed the least to greenhouse gas (GHG) emissions and have the lowest carbon footprints.
- The health-care sector must lead in connecting carbon emissions to health impacts, advocating for adaptive mitigation and resource allocation in vulnerable communities and decarbonization of our own sector.

DEFINITIONS

Climate justice is a concept that addresses the just division, fair sharing, and equitable distribution of both the benefits and burdens of climate change and responsibilities to deal with climate change.

Carbon footprint: Total greenhouse gas (GHG) emissions caused by an individual, event, organization, service, place, or product, expressed as carbon dioxide equivalent (CO_2e)

Allostatic load: Cumulative burden of chronic stress and life events.

Planetary health: A solutions-oriented, transdisciplinary field and social movement focused on analyzing and addressing the impacts of human disruptions to Earth's natural systems on human health and all life on Earth.

Commercial determinants of health (CDoH): The private sector activities affecting public health, either positively or negatively.

Mitigation: Avoiding and reducing GHG emissions through reductions in emissions and sequestration of existing emissions.

Vanderbilt University School of Nursing, 461 21st Avenue South, Nashville, TN 37240, USA
* Corresponding author. Vanderbilt University School of Nursing, 461 21st Avenue South, Frist Hall 364, Nashville, TN 37240.
E-mail address: Carol.c.ziegler@vanderbilt.edu
Twitter: @DrCarolZiegler (C.Z.); @JamesMuturi5 (J.M.)

Prim Care Clin Office Pract 50 (2023) 645–655
https://doi.org/10.1016/j.pop.2023.04.010

Adaptation: The process of adjusting to current or expected effects of climate change.

INTRODUCTION

The World Health Organization has named climate change the greatest threat to human health.[1–3] Globally, ecological impacts from GHG emissions most severely impact the health of communities that have contributed the least to the problem, making climate change an urgent justice issue. Climate justice directly connects to all social determinants of health (SDoH) and social determinants of equity.[4] People with the lowest carbon footprints are most likely to suffer the most severe consequences to their physical and mental well-being, economic insecurity, and community instability due to climate change globally, including in the United States.[5–7] The disproportionate burdens accruing in communities who benefit the least from the profits associated with GHG-emitting activities of industries illuminates the exploitive and complex relationships between SDoH and commercial determinants of health (CDoH). The marked increase in fossil fuel consumption accompanying the industrial revolution created wealth in industrialized nations and for-profit companies and marked the beginning of the shift in atmospheric GHG emissions that have resulted in the current climate crisis.[8] Efforts to reduce GHG emissions for planetary and human health priorities often conflict with the financial and political interests of powerful entities.[9] The health-care industry must lead by example and meaningfully advocate for adaptive mitigation through practice, education, research, and policy advocacy that centers health and climate justice for those disproportionately affected.

Background

Increased accumulation of atmospheric GHG resulting from the burning of fossil fuels for energy causes increases in extreme weather, temperature, and sea level rise.[10] The resulting ecological impacts on our planet directly and significantly influence human and population health and well-being.[2] The goal of the health-care sector, especially primary care, is to provide people with the opportunity to achieve optimal health for as long as possible—to live as well as they can, as long as they can—compressing morbidity to the shortest time possible at the end of life.[11,12] Optimal time on Earth in a healthy state provides increased opportunities for meaningful actions that affect families and communities for generations-like achieving personal fulfillment, accruing intergenerational wealth, investing in rewarding social relationships and building communities. Optimizing health not only "buys time" but also decreases costs (including opportunity costs) to individuals, communities, the health-care system and the nation as a whole.[13]

Ethical concerns connect climate justice and health equity—the equal access to the opportunity to achieve optimal health and its innumerable connected intergenerational benefits. To ensure equitable access to optimal health span in the face of climate change, we must focus on climate justice, integrating adaptation-directed programs while simultaneously mitigating the effects of carbon emissions. The health-care sector is a significant contributor to GHG emissions and must prioritize reaching net zero emissions as soon as possible.[14] This article will explore how climate change contributes to health disparities in vulnerable populations, why this is a justice issue for primary care to address, and what we can do to promote equity, resilience, and adaption in our current economic system while mitigating GHG emissions.

Climate Justice: Who Is Vulnerable?

Geographically, persons in the global south are disproportionately affected by climate change, and in the global north, low-income communities of color and communities with geographic vulnerability are most affected.[7,15] Within the United States and globally, carbon footprint correlates with income level,[15,16] and the individuals and nations who currently and historically contribute the least to carbon emissions suffer the most severe burdens from climate change.[17] Health impacts from climate change are most often and most acutely felt in low-income communities of color.[5,18] Some projections suggest that nations in the global north may benefit from some aspects of climate change, such as prolonged growing seasons, exacerbating current economic inequality between the global north and south.[19,20]

Primary care providers (PCPs) must be able to identify sources of vulnerability and exposure in individuals, families, and communities they care for. As mentioned in the introduction, the health and economic impacts of climate change disproportionately burden people who are already heavily burdened by SDoH and high allostatic load.[18,21–23] When assessing risk, be aware that much of our most granular risk data are based on census tracts and within zip codes; 15-year gaps may exist in life expectancy based on race alone[24]; and these life span gaps perpetuate economic, educational, and health disparities. Additional climate vulnerability may result from personal traits (age, gender); proximity to climate influences such as extreme weather (heat waves, hurricanes, floods, fires, tornadoes, and droughts); or vulnerability to secondary and tertiary impacts such as economic status, social factors, and occupation.[2] People at extremes of age, those exposed to climate impacts through occupational exposure or unsafe housing, and women and people living with comorbidities related to mental and physical health conditions are most vulnerable to the health impacts of climate change.[2,25,26] Occupational exposure poses a significant risk and people whose work or activities leave them exposed to heat, poor air quality, and extreme weather are especially vulnerable.[27] Such workers include outdoor workers, athletes, workers and children in outdoor camps, utility workers, groundskeepers, farmworkers, first responders, and so forth.[27,28] Persons experiencing homelessness or those in unsafe, unhealthy housing are more vulnerable to climate-related health impacts.[7,28,29]

Health Impacts: How These Ecological Impacts Affect Mental and Physical Health

Climate change is projected to impact physical and mental health causing approximately 250, 000 additional deaths between 2030 and 2050, and costing US$2 to US$4 billion per year in direct health-care costs by 2030.[30] Deaths from extreme climatic conditions such as extreme heat waves are now evident—both in high-income and low to middle-income countries—most of the deaths resulting from cardiovascular, kidney and respiratory diseases, and mental illness.[31]

In regards to mental health, the American Psychiatric Association recognizes that climate change poses a significant threat to mental health with a disproportionate burden imposed on children, elderly, and the chronically ill, those with mental illnesses and mobility impairments, and women especially pregnant and postpartum women.[32–35] These mental disorders include posttraumatic stress disorder, depression, anxiety, phobias, sleep disorders, attachment disorders, and substance abuse. In addition to the effects on individual mental health, the possibility of extreme weather and climate disasters creating droughts, flooding, severe storm, tropical cyclone, wildfires, and winter storm may lead to increased conflict and civil strife,[36,37] which significantly challenge mental health of vast populations of people simultaneously. In the best of times, effective mental health resources are very limited, exacerbating existing mental health issues and prolonging time to effective identification and treatment.

In terms of physical health, it is important to note that the root cause of climate change—the burning of fossil fuels—is a major contributor to worldwide mortality through airborne particulate matter and ozone, and ambient air pollution, and is the leading cause of global disease burden in low and middle income countries (LMICs).[38] Fine particulate matter ($PM_{2.5}$) emissions from fossil fuels were estimated to cause 10.2 million global excess deaths in 2012 alone via its cardiac and pulmonary disease impacts.[39] Increasing sea levels, too, can affect physical health, with our current unprecedented increase in temperature,[29] increasing injuries, drowning, and water and soil salinization issues.[40]

The increases in extreme heat, which are now common in the United States and around the globe, can have devastating physical effects—especially in low-resource countries where adequate cooling measures are often unavailable.[41,42] Heat *stroke* is a condition requiring immediate medical attention that occurs from exposure to extreme heat. It occurs when the body temperature increases above 40°C, which if untreated is fatal in 10% to 50% of cases resulting from brain, heart, and kidneys damage.[41] Heat *stress* or heat exhaustion, although less immediate, can cause severe dehydration, acute cerebrovascular accidents, and may contribute to formation of blood clots and other minor manifestations such as lethargy, irritability, headache.[41] In addition, extreme heat compounds the health effects of outdoor air quality by increasing the particulate levels/air pollutants, creating a more serious synergy of air contamination and heat stress, and leading to more serious health harms that those from either alone. People working outdoors are particularly at high risk of heat stress due to increases in core body temperature from muscle activity and the combined effects of heat and humidity.[41]

The world continues to experience several intense climate-related variable weather patterns such as intense heat waves, flooding, droughts, increase in forest fires, tornadoes, and hurricanes. Extreme temperatures are expected to lead to more heat-related illnesses and worsen some chronic medical conditions such as heart disease, respiratory disease, and diabetes.[43,44] At the same time, some medications (such as some antidepressants, diuretics, and beta-blockers) taken for a chronic illness may increase an individual's sensitivity to heat and consequently, people with obesity and heart disease will have at greater risk of heat illnesses or mortality.[44] The climate-related weather changes described above pose humanitarian crises and may lead to civil conflict and forced migration resulting in health-related consequences, psychological distress, risks during pregnancy and childbirth, exposure to violence and discrimination, as well as a lack of adequate health-care services and social support.[45,46] Lessons learnt from global terrorism and recent pandemics should gear us to prepare for potential risks developing from climate change. Despite the overwhelming evidence and lessons learnt from other threats, there is still underinvestment and unpreparedness in public health measures and health systems preparation to address climate change and subsequent large-scale health impacts.

Stress: Allostatic Load, Climate, and Economic Impacts

Allostatic load ensues when environmental challenges exceed the individual's ability to cope. Allostatic load reflects a cumulative effect of stressful experiences in daily life including climate stress, work stress, behavioral factors such as poor sleep, sedentary lifestyle, smoking, alcohol, or unhealthy diet, as well as major life alterations such as death of loved ones or forced migration.[47] Accumulative evidence from epidemiological, genomic, and other biological studies show that experiences in the natural environment or environmental degradation influence physiology and behavior, which may lead to deleterious health effects.[47] With the increasing occurrences of natural and climate-related environmental disasters, the world has seen devastating costs to both human well-being and economic functioning. The increased allostatic load accumulating from climate disasters has a significant toll on health. As we continue to see billion-dollar environmental disasters (in 2020–2021, the US recorded 42 such events[48] and globally, such disasters have increased 1.7 fold in the last decade), the allostatic load imposed will continue to exert its toll, being, in part, responsible for an increase of 1.23 million deaths, and more than 4 billion people's economic losses.[49]

The Impact of Climate on Social Determinants of Health

Increased heat, extreme weather, and sea level rise and the subsequent far-reaching community impacts touch each of the SDoH, and although the direct economic and health influences of climate change are clear, establishing direct links between climate change and educational access, social and community context, and the built environment is more complex, and more research needs to be done in these areas. In addition to economic devastation and health impacts, extreme weather events such as tornadoes, hurricanes, and flooding may simultaneously and for extended periods of time destroy the built environment and disrupt community context as well as educational access. Not only are structures affected but also families may be displaced. It is important to note that renters are often unable to access Federal Emergency Management Assistance and also are not included in home buyout programs in managed retreat scenarios, leaving them with extensive losses in climate disasters.[50,51]

Heat poses a unique risk in urban communities due to the urban heat island effect, in which the decreased vegetation and increased concrete further exacerbates heat and also diminishes night time cooling—a key protective factor for heat-related morbidity in households without air conditioning.[41,52] Compounding this impact, in many communities, there is no requirement for air conditioning in public housing leaving the underserved especially vulnerable to heat-induced health issues.

Climate Change in the Clinical Encounter

In the clinical encounter, PCPs can assess climate-related risks and promote adaptation and resilience in the following ways: (1) Be aware of local/regional climate vulnerabilities, that is, temperature, extreme weather, and so forth. (2) Assess patients' individual risk and vulnerabilities including baseline physical and mental health, occupation, and environmental risk and exposures. (3) Specifically assess access to safe and healthy housing and temperature control and refer for air conditioning assistance programs and home energy retrofit assistance programs for those who are eligible. (4) Educate patients about heat and air-quality indices and how to adjust behaviors to optimize health based on their individual risk. (5) Talk to patients about safety planning and emergency preparedness for extreme weather and extreme heat and share information about passive cooling techniques. (6) Assess food security and dietary habits and educate patients about optimal diet and hydration status. (7) Optimize management of chronic conditions and ensure preventive care and vaccinations are up to date.

Promoting Cobenefits

Providers can also advocate for cobenefits in the clinical setting. Cobenefits align carbon mitigation with health-promoting activities, and integrating these priorities into education, practice, research, and policy aligns the agendas of planetary and human health. *Project Drawdown* cites the top 100 ways to mitigate GHG[53] and *Nurses*

Drawdown[54] outlines attainable cobenefits with adaptive mitigation for health-care providers. Promoting plant-based diets improves health and reduces GHG emissions from foods[55,56] and the Planetary Health Diet aligns closely with the Mediterranean diet,[57] ideal for reducing cardiovascular risk. Increased life span, decreased cardiovascular and cancer risk, as well as avoided carbon emissions are cobenefits of such diets.[14,57,58] Access to gardens for locally sourced produce, as well as green space and tree cover, promotes health and well-being on multiple fronts[59] and sequesters GHG.[60–62] Certain trees improve air quality and reduce respiratory illness.[63–65] Food waste is a significant source of carbon emissions and dietary interventions to increase plant-based diets, reduce wasteful consumption, eliminate food waste, and promote composting result in decreased GHG emissions.[66,67] Home energy retrofit assistance programs for low-income home owners and the elderly have been shown to improve health measures, decrease financial burdens from utility bill reductions, and decrease emissions from utilities.[68] Advocating for and utilizing all of these strategies is within the scope of the primary care clinician (Appendix).

Maximizing Resilience and Promoting Mitigation: Advocacy from the Health-Care Sector

The health-care sector must integrate climate justice principles in policy, research, education, and practice. We have social credibility, public trust, economic purchasing power, and political power. Gallup ranks nurses as the most trusted profession for the 21st year in a row, followed by medical doctors, and we are crucial voices in addressing climate justice and promoting planetary health.[69] We are the world's frontline health-care providers as well as the most trusted professionals, and our advocacy is powerful.

Intentionally elevate leadership of indigenous communities and communities of color. To effectively shift our metaparadigm grounded and founded in colonial ways of being, we have to think beyond mitigation and adaptation to envision a new global community and invite and center the voices of leaders who will lead efforts to decolonize our ways of thinking and being and promote planetary health.[70–73] Meaningfully inclusive practices promote the types of disruptive innovation and radical collaboration that will usher in creative practice models, and justice-centered policies. Educate yourself about decolonizing health care and advocate for these practices in your institutions.

Achieve net zero emissions within the health-care sector. If the global health-care sector were a country, it would be the 13th largest emitter of GHGs in the world.[14] In the United States, the health-care sector accounts for 18% of our GDP and contributes 10% of our GHG emissions.[14] The sources of these emissions are supply chain (pharmaceuticals, chemicals, food, and so forth at roughly 70%), purchased power (at roughly 11%), and direct emissions (from things such as anesthesia.).[14] Tertiary care is expensive and carbon intensive, and there is a correlation between per capita GHG emissions and health-care expenditures.[14] Transparency, mandatory emissions reporting and regulated accountability must be embedded into reimbursement formulas and institutional accreditation in addition to increased investments in primary care[14] and support for the recent call to sign on to the fossil fuel nonproliferation treaty.[74] Institutions and professional organizations must lobby for clean energy, clean transportation and just renewable transitions, account for the carbon emissions of transportation for patient visits as well as professional activities and conferences, and prioritize low carbon practices such as telemedicine and web-based conferences.[75–77]

SUMMARY

Climate change is the greatest threat to human health today. The root cause of climate change, fossil fuel emissions, also contributes significantly to the top 100 causes of death globally. Therefore, transitioning to clean energy improves health and promotes climate justice.

CLINICS CARE POINTS

- Low-income families contribute the least to carbon emissions yet bear the greatest health and financial burdens associated with climate change.
- Heat exposure, respiratory conditions from poor air quality, vector and allergen-borne illnesses, injuries from extreme weather events, and mental health impacts are climate-related health issues that primary care providers must be aware of and prepared to manage.
- Climate education and planetary health must be integrated in education across all health-related fields and required for continued licensure certification.
- Health-care sector emissions are a significant contributor to climate change and achieving net zero emissions as a sector must be prioritized.

DISCLOSURE

The authors have nothing to disclose.

SUPPLEMENTARY DATA

Supplementary data related to this article can be found online at https://doi.org/10.1016/j.pop.2023.04.010.

REFERENCES

1. Ziegler C, Morelli V, Fawibe O. Climate Change and Underserved Communities. Prim Care Clin Off Pract 2017;44(1):171–84.
2. Ziegler C, Morelli V, Fawibe O. Climate change and underserved communities. Physician Assist Clin 2019;4(1):203–16.
3. World Health Organization. Regional Office for the Eastern Mediterranean. (↱2005)↱. Address by Dr Hussein A. Gezairy, Regional Director, WHO Eastern Mediterranean Region, to the regional consultation on the role of social determinants in improving health outcomes, Cairo, Egypt, 8-9 May 2005. Available at: https://apps.who.int/iris/handle/10665/126080.
4. Marmot M, Allen JJ. Social determinants of health equity. Am J Public Health 2014;104(S4):S517–9.
5. Levy BS, Patz JA. Climate change, human rights, and social justice. Ann Glob Health 2015;81(3):310–22.
6. Islam N, Winkel J, "Climate Change and Social Inequality", *UN Department of Economic and Social Affairs (DESA) Working Papers*, No. 152, UN, New York, 2017. Available at: https://doi.org/10.18356/2c62335d-en.
7. Shonkoff S, Morello-Frosch R, Pastor M, et al. The climate gap: Environmental health and equity implications of climate change and mitigation policies in California—A review of the literature. Climatic Change 2012;109:485–503. https://doi.org/10.1007/s10584-011-0310-7.

8. Martinez LH. Post industrial revolution human activity and climate change: Why The United States must implement mandatory limits on industrial greenhouse gas emmissions. J Land Use Environ Law 2005;403–21.
9. Hansen T. Stranded assets and reduced profits: Analyzing the economic underpinnings of the fossil fuel industry's resistance to climate stabilization. Renew Sustain Energy Rev 2022;158:112144.
10. Yoro KO, Daramola MO. CO2 emission sources, greenhouse gases, and the global warming effect. In: Advances in carbon Capture. Elsevier; 2020. p. 3–28.
11. Crimmins EM. Lifespan and healthspan: past, present, and promise. Gerontol 2015;55(6):901–11.
12. Partridge L, Deelen J, Slagboom PE. Facing up to the global challenges of ageing. Nature 2018;561(7721):45–56.
13. Semenza JC. Climate change and human health. Int J Environ Res Public Health 2014;11(7):7347–53.
14. Eckelman MJ, Sherman J. Environmental impacts of the US health care system and effects on public health. PLoS One 2016;11(6):e0157014.
15. Goldstein B, Gounaridis D, Newell JP. The carbon footprint of household energy use in the United States. Proc Natl Acad Sci 2020;117(32):19122–30.
16. Bruckner B, Hubacek K, Shan Y, et al. Impacts of poverty alleviation on national and global carbon emissions. Nat Sustain 2022;5(4):311–20.
17. Kennedy EH, Krahn H, Krogman NT. Egregious emitters: Disproportionality in household carbon footprints. Environ Behav 2014;46(5):535–55.
18. Gasper R, Blohm A, Ruth M. Social and economic impacts of climate change on the urban environment. Curr Opin Environ Sustain 2011;3(3):150–7.
19. Puaschunder JM. Climate in the 21st century: a macroeconomic model of fair global warming benefits distribution to grant climate justice around the world and over time. In: ; 2018.
20. Diffenbaugh NS, Burke M. Global warming has increased global economic inequality. Proc Natl Acad Sci 2019;116(20):9808–13.
21. Robinette JW, Charles ST, Almeida DM, et al. Neighborhood features and physiological risk: An examination of allostatic load. Health Place 2016;41:110–8.
22. Blair C, Raver CC, Granger D, et al. Family Life Project Key Investigators. Allostasis and allostatic load in the context of poverty in early childhood. Dev Psychopathol 2011;23(3):845–57.
23. Schulz AJ, Mentz G, Lachance L, et al. Associations between socioeconomic status and allostatic load: effects of neighborhood poverty and tests of mediating pathways. Am J Public Health 2012;102(9):1706–14.
24. Dwyer-Lindgren L, Kendrick P, Kelly YO, et al. Life expectancy by county, race, and ethnicity in the USA, 2000–19: a systematic analysis of health disparities. Lancet 2022;400(10345):25–38.
25. Haines A, Kovats RS, Campbell-Lendrum D, et al. Climate change and human health: impacts, vulnerability and public health. Publ Health 2006;120(7):585–96.
26. McMichael AJ, Haines J, Slooff R, et al, World Health Organization. Climate change and human health: an assessment/prepared by a Task Group on behalf of the World Health Organization, the World Meteorological Association and the United Nations Environment Programme; editors: AJ McMichael. et al. In: Climate Change and Human Health: An Assessment/Prepared by a Task Group on Behalf of the World Health Organization, the World Meteorological Association and the United Nations Environment Programme; Editors:. ; 1996.
27. Applebaum KM, Graham J, Gray GM, et al. An overview of occupational risks from climate change. Curr Environ Health Rep 2016;3:13–22.

28. Schulte PA, Chun H. Climate change and occupational safety and health: establishing a preliminary framework. J Occup Environ Hyg 2009;6(9):542–54.
29. Meierrieks D. Weather shocks, climate change and human health. World Dev 2021;138:105228.
30. World Health Organization. Climate change and health. Published October 30, 2022. Accessed January 24, 2023. https://www.who.int/news-room/fact-sheets/detail/climate-change-and-health.
31. Centers for Disease Control and Prevention. Climate Effects on Health. Published April 25, 2022. Accessed January 24, 2023. https://www.cdc.gov/climateandhealth/effects/default.htm.
32. Ursano RJ, Morganstein JC, Cooper R. APA Resource Document: Resource Document on Mental Health and Climate Change. Published online 2017. Accessed January 24, 2022. https://www.psychiatry.org/File%20Library/Psychiatrists/Directories/Library-and-Archive/resource_documents/2017-Resource-Document-Mental-Health-Climate-Change.pdf.
33. Xiong X, Harville EW, Mattison DR, et al. Hurricane Katrina experience and the risk of post-traumatic stress disorder and depression among pregnant women. Am J Disaster Med 2010;5(3):181–7. https://doi.org/10.5055/ajdm.2010.0020.
34. Bei B, Bryant C, Gilson KM, et al. A prospective study of the impact of floods on the mental and physical health of older adults. Aging Ment Health 2013;17(8):992–1002. https://doi.org/10.1080/13607863.2013.799119.
35. Burke SEL, Sanson AV, Van Hoorn J. The Psychological Effects of Climate Change on Children. Curr Psychiatry Rep 2018;20(5):35. https://doi.org/10.1007/s11920-018-0896-9.
36. Ministry of Health. National strategic plan for prevention and control of NCDs 2020/21-2025/26. 2021. Available at: https://www.health.go.ke/wp-content/uploads/2021/07/Kenya-Non-Communicable-Disease-NCD-Strategic-Plan-2021-2025.pdf. Accessed December 12, 2022.
37. Balsari S, Dresser C, Leaning J. Climate Change, Migration, and Civil Strife. Curr Environ Health Rep 2020;7(4):404–14.
38. Forouzanfar Mohammad H, Afshin Ashkan, Alexander Lily T, et al. Global, regional, and national comparative risk assessment of 79 behavioural, environmental and occupational, and metabolic risks or clusters of risks, 1990–2015: a systematic analysis for the Global Burden of Disease Study 2015. Lancet 2016;388(10053):1659–724.
39. Vohra K, Vodonos A, Schwartz J, et al. Global mortality from outdoor fine particle pollution generated by fossil fuel combustion: Results from GEOS-Chem. Environ Res 2021;195:110754.
40. Mazhar S, Pellegrini E, Contin M, et al. Impacts of salinization caused by sea level rise on the biological processes of coastal soils - A review. Front Environ Sci. 2022;10. Accessed March 3, 2023. https://www.frontiersin.org/articles/10.3389/fenvs.2022.909415.
41. Howard S, Krishna G. How hot weather kills: the rising public health dangers of extreme heat. BMJ 2022;378:o1741.
42. Parkes B, Buzan JR, Huber M. Heat stress in Africa under high intensity climate change. Int J Biometeorol 2022;66(8):1531–45. https://doi.org/10.1007/s00484-022-02295-1.
43. Sarofim MC, Saha S, Hawkins MD, et al. Ch. 2: temperature-related death and illness. The impacts of climate change on human health in the United States: a Scientific Assessment. U.S. Global Change Research Program; 2016. p. 43–68.

https://doi.org/10.7930/J0MG7MDX. Available at: https://health2016.globalchange.gov/temperature-related-death-and-illness. Available at:.
44. United States Environmental Protection Agency. Climate Change and the Health of People with Chronic Medical Conditions. Accessed March 3, 2023. https://www.epa.gov/climateimpacts/climate-change-and-health-people-chronic-medical-conditions#28foot.
45. Mazhin SA, Khankeh H, Farrokhi M, et al. Migration health crisis associated with climate change: A systematic review. J Educ Health Promot 2020;9:97. https://doi.org/10.4103/jehp.jehp_4_20.
46. Jolof L, Rocca P, Mazaheri M, et al. Experiences of armed conflicts and forced migration among women from countries in the Middle East, Balkans, and Africa: a systematic review of qualitative studies. Confl Health 2022;16(1):46. https://doi.org/10.1186/s13031-022-00481-x.
47. Logan AC, Prescott SL, Haahtela T, et al. The importance of the exposome and allostatic load in the planetary health paradigm. J Physiol Anthropol 2018;37(1):15. https://doi.org/10.1186/s40101-018-0176-8.
48. National Oceanic and Atmospheric Administration. Billion-Dollar Weather and Climate Disasters. Published 2023. Accessed January 26, 2023. https://www.ncei.noaa.gov/access/billions/.
49. Centre for Research on the Epidemiology of Disasters. UNISDR and CRED report: economic losses, Poverty & disasters (1998 - 2017). Published 2018. Accessed January 26, 2023. https://www.cred.be/unisdr-and-cred-report-economic-losses-poverty-disasters-1998-2017.
50. Dundon LA, Camp JS. Climate justice and home-buyout programs: renters as a forgotten population in managed retreat actions. J Environ Stud Sci 2021;11(3):420–33.
51. Drakes O, Tate E, Rainey J, et al. Social vulnerability and short-term disaster assistance in the United States. Int J Disaster Risk Reduct 2021;53:102010.
52. He C, Kim H, Hashizume M, et al. The effects of night-time warming on mortality burden under future climate change scenarios: a modelling study. Lancet Planet Health 2022;6(8):e648–57.
53. Tegler B. Drawdown: The Most Comprehensive Plan Ever Proposed to Reverse Global Warming" by Paul Hawken, 2016.[book review]. Can Field Nat 2017;131(2):197.
54. Huffling K. Nurses Drawdown: Building a Nurse-Led, Solutions-Based Quality Improvement Project to Address Climate Change. Creat Nurs 2021;27(4):245–50.
55. Springmann M, Wiebe K, Mason-D'Croz D, et al. Health and nutritional aspects of sustainable diet strategies and their association with environmental impacts: a global modelling analysis with country-level detail. Lancet Planet Health 2018;2(10):e451–61.
56. Gibbs J, Cappuccio FP. Plant-based dietary patterns for human and planetary health. Nutrients 2022;14(8):1614.
57. Verschuren WM, Boer JM, Temme EH. Optimal diet for cardiovascular and planetary health. Heart 2022;108(15):1234–9.
58. Frumkin H. The US health care sector's carbon footprint: stomping or treading lightly? Am J Public Health 2018;108(S2):S56–7.
59. Barron S, Nitoslawski S, Wolf KL, et al. Greening blocks: A conceptual typology of practical design interventions to integrate health and climate resilience co-benefits. Int J Environ Res Public Health 2019;16(21):4241.
60. Renforth P, Edmondson J, Leake JR, et al. Designing a carbon capture function into urban soils. Proc Inst Civ Eng-Urban Des Plan 2011;164(2):121–8.

61. Guo Z, Zhang Z, Wu X, et al. Building shading affects the ecosystem service of urban green spaces: Carbon capture in street canyons. Ecol Model 2020;431: 109178.
62. Shadman S, Khalid PA, Hanafiah MM, et al. The carbon sequestration potential of urban public parks of densely populated cities to improve environmental sustainability. Sustain Energy Technol Assess 2022;52:102064.
63. Nowak DJ, McPherson EG. Quantifying the impact of trees: The Chicago urban forest climate project. Unasylva 1993;173(44):39–44.
64. Lai Y, Kontokosta CE. The impact of urban street tree species on air quality and respiratory illness: A spatial analysis of large-scale, high-resolution urban data. Health Place 2019;56:80–7.
65. Beckett KP, Freer Smith P, Taylor G. Effective tree species for local air quality management. Arboric J 2000;26(1):12–9.
66. Mariam N, Valerie K, Karin D, et al. Limiting food waste via grassroots initiatives as a potential for climate change mitigation: a systematic review. Environ Res Lett 2020;15(12):123008.
67. Chapagain A, James K. Accounting for the impact of food waste on water resources and climate change. Food Ind Wastes 2013;217–36.
68. Tonn B, Hawkins B, Rose E, et al. Income, housing and health: Poverty in the United States through the prism of residential energy efficiency programs. Energy Res Soc Sci 2021;73:101945.
69. Kurth A, Potter T. The Public Health Crisis Is Planetary—and Nursing Is Crucial to Addressing It. Am J Public Health 2022;112(S3):S259–61.
70. Redvers N. The value of global indigenous knowledge in planetary health. Challenges 2018;9(2):30.
71. Redvers N. The determinants of planetary health. Lancet Planet Health 2021;5(3): e111–2.
72. Redvers N, Poelina A, Schultz C, et al. Indigenous natural and first law in planetary health. Challenges 2020;11(2):29.
73. Redvers N, Celidwen Y, Schultz C, et al. The determinants of planetary health: an Indigenous consensus perspective. Lancet Planet Health 2022;6(2):e156–63.
74. Howard C, Beagley J, Eissa M, et al. Why we need a fossil fuel non-proliferation treaty. Lancet Planet Health 2022;6(10):e777–8.
75. Purohit A, Smith J, Hibble A. Does telemedicine reduce the carbon footprint of healthcare? A systematic review. Future Healthc J 2021;8(1):e85.
76. Zotova O, Pétrin-Desrosiers C, Gopfert A, et al. Carbon-neutral medical conferences should be the norm. Lancet Planet Health 2020;4(2):e48–50.
77. Roberts I, Godlee F. Reducing the carbon footprint of medical conferences. BMJ 2007;334(7589):324–5.

The Digital Domain

A "Super" Social Determinant of Health

Rachel Hanebutt, EdM, MA*, Hasina Mohyuddin, PhD

KEYWORDS

• Digital health • Telehealth • Digital equity and inclusion • Broadband access
• Digital literacy

KEY POINTS

- The digital divide—or disparities between those with digital access and know-how and those without—continues to disproportionately influence marginalized populations in the United States; these groups tend to also be marginalized by the health care system.
- Digital access and connectivity are essential for all aspects of health care today, including patient-provider communication, patient accessibility to care, and health care quality.
- Different patient populations have different needs when it comes to health care; this reality is also true for learning to use and leverage digital health interventions and digital communication strategies that are tied to the patient-provider relationship.
- Primary care physicians can play an important role in the adoption of digital technologies, as well as increasing digital skills, to increase digital health equity.

INTRODUCTION

There is no question that access to the Internet has become necessary for thriving in today's society, as the impact of the digital domain extends to all areas of life, including individual, family, and community health outcomes. This reality is especially true for patient-provider relationships, as access to and the use of digital tools within medical and health care settings (eg, patient portals, health monitoring devices, and apps) is constantly evolving.[1] Further, *The Lancet and Financial Times Commission On Governing Health Futures 2030: Growing Up in a Digital World* argued that digital transformations—including digital health interventions, using technology to advance health, and digital equity—should be considered a key determinant of health.[2] This article presents the case of the digital domain as a "super" social determinant of health and provides a primer of key insight for primary care providers regarding their

Department of Human and Organizational Development, Vanderbilt University Peabody College, Nashville, TN, USA
* Corresponding author. 230 Appleton Pl #5721, Nashville, TN, 37203, USA
E-mail address: rachel.a.hanebutt@vanderbilt.edu

Prim Care Clin Office Pract 50 (2023) 657–670
https://doi.org/10.1016/j.pop.2023.04.002

individual and collective roles within the context of creating an infrastructure of equitable digital access in order to achieve health equity for all.

HISTORY

Historically, health care has always been marked by advances in technology, and digital technologies now affect nearly all aspects of the health care delivery system.[3] However, the focus has typically been on how advances in technology might be used by health care providers to improve diagnosis and treatment, rather than on how it might be used by patients. In considering the use of technology from the patient perspective, though, we can see how advancements in digital technologies can shift the ways in which health care is perceived and consumed by individuals. From the first recorded instance of a telemedicine visit—which occurred in 1897 when a child was diagnosed with croup during a telephone consultation with a physician[4]—to the present day, technology has proved its ability to improve patient access to information and services. Although the increasing use of the telephone allowed for consultations with physicians for those in remote areas, telephone-based consultation with a primary care provider has had limitations for overall quality of care.[5] It was not until the latter half of the twentieth century that the growth of digital health care became much more prevalent. The early days of the Internet allowed individuals greater access to health information and ushered in the age of Dr. Google or increased patient reliance on online information for making health care decisions. It also created connection opportunities and specifically, the opportunity to learn more about health care providers, insurance benefits, and other aspects of health care delivery to improve the choices that individuals were able to make about their own health.[6] Further, the founding of several professional associations such as the American Telemedicine Association and the International Medical Informatics Association worked to improve the use of digital communication in health care delivery. The twenty-first century, then, saw advancements in technological innovations, such as the emergence of digital health portals, apps, and wearable devices (such as the Fitbit and Apple Watch) that further allowed individuals to be agentic in how they approached health care. However, not all individuals were able to reap the benefits of these advancements in technology, as digital access remained elusive for many.

The COVID-19 pandemic exacerbated digital access issues, especially for low-income, Black, and Latinx communities who were financially strained and forced to stop their home Internet subscriptions.[7] The ability to schedule an appointment online in order to receive a vaccine was also implicated by digital equity. It is important to note that the influence of the COVID-19 pandemic on digital access is bidirectional. According to Early and Hernandez (2021), "Digital disenfranchisement, racism, and other structural barriers faced by communities of color have contributed to devastating loss of life from COVID-19" (pg. 607). In other words, the lack of digital access can sometimes lead to the loss of life. However, the changing nature of patient-provider relationships during the pandemic also highlighted the role that telehealth can have in increasing access to services for these underserved communities. To expand on this history, the next section provides key definitions pertinent to the digital domain and health care.

DEFINITIONS

The following definitions are especially beneficial for primary care physicians and health care professionals, as they directly outline the key aspects of the digital domain that influence patient health.

- *Digital Access vs. Digital Adoption* is a debate within digital inclusion conversations wherein simply ensuring digital access does not necessitate digital adoption: digital access does not imply Internet or device use. In other words, digital adoption focuses on the willingness of individuals and communities to access and use digital technologies to their personal benefit, whereas digital access stops short by focusing on the goal of access to the Internet and devices.
- *Digital Equity* is the goal of many digital inclusion efforts, which includes creating a more equitable society in which all people have equitable access, opportunity, and know-how to benefit from the digital world. Given that many "made-to-be-minorized" communities—or those affected by the imposition of larger, structural forces that actively put some into disadvantaged societal realities while privileging others based on social class, race, or other factors—are already underserved by the health care system, the influence of equitable digital access, devices, and skills has a compounded impact on these populations and their health.
- *Digital Disenfranchisement* is being deprived of one's right to access, operate, and use digital technology in service of their own livelihood and well-being. Recent studies have found evidence that digital disenfranchisement exacerbates and contributes a variety of negative health outcomes, racial injustices, and economic oppression, as well as other social determinants of health (eg, education, food security). The framing of digital disenfranchisement appropriately positions access to the digital domain as an important health advocacy issue (see later discussion).[8]
- *Digital Health Literacy* involves the application of one's cognitive and social abilities to access, understand, and use health information within digital contexts and environments with a goal of learning about, addressing, or solving a health problem. Digital health literacy has been defined as a super determinant of health (see later discussion).[9,10]
- *Digital Inclusion* is the practice and process of providing all individuals and communities with access to high-quality broadband Internet, affordable and adequate Internet-enabled devices, and the necessary support for digital skills training to become digitally literate. Thus, digital inclusion for primary care providers focuses on ensuring accessible digital systems (eg, electronic health records [EHRs]), communication (eg, telehealth or telemedicine appointments), and support (eg, accessible digital communication) that enhance their ability to provide patients with high-quality, patient-focused care.
- *Telehealth* broadly concerns any technology-related health technology and the delivery of health care services, including telemedicine (eg, virtual appointments with doctors). The aim of telehealth is to increase the accessibility to health care and health information; this is of particular concern for patients living in underserved communities (ie, rural, remote areas) without adequate or equitable health care facilities, which could include consultations with one's doctor, treatments, or communication provided via remote communication technologies (eg, video conferencing, telephones, etc.). It is often used interchangeably with telemedicine, although telemedicine refers specifically to remote access of clinical care, whereas telehealth may sometimes encompass a broader scope of health care services, such as provider training.

BACKGROUND

According to the Pew Research Center, 1 out of every 4 American adults do not have access to broadband Internet, and 7% of Americans report not using the Internet.[11]

These estimates do not even include millions of Americans who are underconnected or lack a stable Internet connection to use the Internet in basic ways. In addition, self-reported coverage data from Internet service providers might underestimate the number of people without adequate or affordable access.[12] Unpacking the broadband equation is important because access is now a "basic need" within our increasingly digital society, as the Internet has the capacity to connect people to employment and educational opportunities, food, information, and even health care.[8]

By definition, social determinants of health are "conditions in the places where people live, learn, work, and play that affect a wide range of health and quality-of-life-risks and outcomes."[13] The digital domain has been called a "super" determinant of health due to the ways in which digital literacy and Internet connectivity influence a multitude of other areas of life and health.[14] The other areas influenced by digital literacy and access include economic sustainability (eg, medical bills, employment, online shopping), neighborhood and physical environment (eg, finding housing, transportation), education (eg, literacy, vocational training opportunities), food (eg, finding and using safety net program access, fresh food access, and delivery), community and social context (eg, social support systems, community engagement, access to news and information), and of course, the health care system (eg, finding health coverage, using telehealth, health apps, and patient portals).[15] Although each of these aspects warrant its own investigation, the health care system's relationship with the digital divide has a more direct influence on health, with the patient-provider relationship serving as one of the most central components to the reasons that digital domain influences health. For example, patients with certain types of health conditions, such as mental health issues, may have inequitable social determinants of health but may be more likely to use digital platforms and services if a good patient-provider relationship has been established.[16] This fact further elevates the importance of this article.

To systematically address the digital domain as a social determinant of health, we will consider the core issues of digital equity—digital access, digital devices, and digital skills and literacy—and the implications each have for health more broadly. Importantly, each section of the discussion focuses on key considerations for the patient-provider relationship, as direct patient care is the focus of this handbook.

DISCUSSION

To start, equity within the digital domain is not confined to health care or dependent on primary care providers to ensure that all patients have the access, knowledge, and skills that they need to thrive in the digital world. However, it is essential that physicians and primary care teams are well versed in the ways that the digital domain manifests as a social determinant of health. As such, it is essential that physicians understand the following: (1) that digital inequities and exclusion, in general, are social determinants of health; (2) how *digital access*, or access to high-quality broadband affects health care and health outcomes; (3) how *device access and use* (and nonuse) affect health care and health outcomes; and (4) how *digital skills and literacies* influence patient health. In addition to these 4, broad but important aspects of the digital domain, additional considerations central to the patient-provider relationship are considered (ie, patient health advocacy and community engagement). These key areas are described in more detail in the sections that follow.

Digital Equity and Inclusion and Social Determinants of Health

Just as health equity provides an essential framework for ensuring that all people receive the health care, digital equity overarches all aspects of the digital world, advocating that individuals and communities have the right to access, operate, and use digital technology in the service of their own livelihood and well-being. Putting these 2 important ideas together, Richardson and colleagues' (2022) framework for digital health equity goes as far as to frame the social determinants of health within the digital domain as *digital* determinants of health, existing at all levels of the socio-ecological model with implications that extend past the digital realm, as well as beyond the health care realm.[17] Although it does not have a single or fixed definition, the National Digital Inclusion Alliance (NDIA), a community of digital inclusion practitioners and advocates, broadly paints digital inclusion, as "the activities necessary to ensure that all individuals and communities, including the most disadvantaged, have access to and use of information and communication technologies."[18] In this sense, *digital inclusion* represents a set of practices and efforts to ensure that all individuals have access to and a complete understanding of the digital domain, with *digital equity* being the goal wherein this is a reality for all individuals, regardless of their background, social standing, or health.

Even though there are numerous federal and state efforts to increase *access* to digital technologies to communities, there may still be reasons why individuals might not choose to *adopt* those technologies—from worries about security and privacy to lack of comfort using the Internet or digital devices; this is referred to as the digital access versus digital adoption debate: although important, digital access is just part of the equation for getting individuals and families online. There is space within this debate for primary care physicians to play an important role in the increased adoption of digital technology, particularly for underserved communities. For many patients in such communities, primary care providers are trusted professionals whose expertise is valued. Patient education efforts that occur within the patient-provider dynamic are a form of digital inclusion that can affect other aspects of an individual's well-being (ie, economic, transportation, nutrition), in addition to health and health equity. In sum, providing patients with an understanding of how adoption of digital technologies might positively affect their health outcomes has been shown to be beneficial for enhancing health-related outcomes, as discussed in more detail in the sections that follow.

Digital Access as a Social Determinant of Health

As with most aspects of our digital world, digital access is oftentimes the first step of engagement and a natural entry point for digital experiences and advancement. According to the Federal Communications Commission (FCC) National Broadband Map, nearly all United States residents had access to at least 1 Internet service provider in 2021; however, 10 million people—including those living in rural communities and two-thirds of tribal communities—still did not have sufficient access to high-speed Internet.[19] Given that these statistics often rely on self-reported data, it should also be assumed that there is a greater divide between those who have consistent, high-quality broadband Internet with adequate download speeds and those who do not.[12]

Of particular concern to primary care providers, "digitally isolated communities may risk worse health outcomes resulting from the effects of limited broadband access on educational and economic opportunities as well as access to high-quality health services."[20(p41)] In addition, one's ability to access high-quality broadband depends on the laws and procedures of their state or municipality. Regardless of location or context, broadband Internet access has been proposed to accompany "information" as an overriding influence of social determinants of health, as recognized by the American Medical Association. From this perspective, digital access has influence on the health care system, economic stability, food, education, community and social context, and neighborhood and physical environment, all of which affect key health outcomes (eg, mortality, morbidity, life expectancy, and so forth).[21] The far-reaching influence of digital access can be best understood by understanding the following areas: (1) how patients *access and navigate the healthcare system* via their digital access; (2) how patients are *engaged and educated* by providers via their digital access; and (3) how patients leverage and act on health insights based on *telehealth* and subsequent *health behaviors*. This last point is important to emphasize, as digital access requires not only access and adoption but an active behavioral aspect to be fully used for advancing patient health.

Health care access and navigation

The digital domain enables patients additional and extended opportunities to use online platforms to find, compare, and select health care providers and services, thereby improving their access to health care overall. Digital access has also enabled sharing of EHRs within patient portals, which have become a gateway to other health applications and platform use. Lack of access then compounds inequalities when patients are not able to access or use these systems.[22] The adoption of smartphones with data plans has helped to close the digital divide, increasing patient access to EHRs and patient portals; however, there are still equity, privacy, and ethical concerns when assuming that all patients have access to the health portals they need.[23] Publicly available methods for accessing health information—such as public Wi-Fi and libraries—may not be comfortable or preferred by patients who are conscious of their data privacy and safety. According to the American Library Association, many libraries are not bound to HIPAA regulations that protect user data, leaving patients' data privacy and security dependent on library resources, priorities, and sometimes location-based legal regulations.[24] However, this risk to health data security should not undermine the value that health science and public libraries and librarians have for increasing methods for all patients to access critical health information online.[25] Whether it be via home access or another avenue, understanding how patients are able to access online health care systems is an essential first step for providers seeking to use these important technologies.

Health engagement and education

Accessing patient portals and platforms is just part of the digital access equation. Another key aspect includes *how* patients engage with these online systems, which is wrought with its own set of barriers. Specifically, a review of patient access of digital health records within inpatient settings revealed that lack of portal design and testing and individual patient challenges (eg, doubt of portal usefulness, lost passwords, difficulty in navigating portal, patient anxiety with viewing personal medical information, and lack of encouragement from providers to use portals) were key barriers in using digital health records.[26] Further, the same review found improving patient-provider communication around and within portal use, improving accuracy and timeliness of record keeping, and explicit provider encouragement to be facilitators of patient portal use. When it comes to patient education, past research indicates that patients who receive education materials that are individualized to their own learning style preference and health literacy level showed greater gains in health-related knowledge and even achieved greater levels of disease management and behavior change goals.[27]

Although these examples focus on patient health portals specifically, lessons surrounding the role of platform design and encouragement of use have serious implications for patients' views of the value and importance of digitally accessing their health information and in turn, influences how they engage with these systems. In other words, patient education and encouragement surrounding digital access is essential for adoption of these important health practices.

Telehealth and related health behaviors

We have highlighted the role providers can play to support patient navigation of digital access and engagement with the digital access points related to their health; however, a third piece of this puzzle includes actual use of telehealth and health behavior change resulting from this access; this is especially important for patients with limited access to the Internet, disabilities, limited English proficiency, low digital literacy, and those who are elderly, who may not be as well versed in telehealth practices or the behaviors needed to receive care in this way.[28] In addition, there is currently a lack of consensus in defining telehealth, as "clear definitions of available telehealth services, though they may not solve all forms of inequity, have the potential to reduce misunderstandings, miscommunications, and confusion, all of which contribute to a lack of access to telehealth services."[29(p3)] For the purposes of this article, we have defined telehealth as, "any technology-related health technology and the delivery of health care services," with the assumption that telehealth technologies share a goal of improved patient health outcomes. As mentioned earlier, accessing telehealth is also a digital access concern, as broadband adoption or usage for telehealth relies on patient understanding and behavioral characteristics. Importantly, the COVID-19 pandemic increased usage and awareness of telehealth options and needs across the country, extending current telehealth options beyond just rural and underserved settings.[30]

Telehealth options are comparable to traditional, in-person visits, as it pertains to patient satisfaction and engagement and patient-provider communication.[31,32] However, qualitative insight of primary care practice models that specifically leverage virtual patient visits for rural patients found that empowering asynchronous communication and leveraging virtual care were valuable for practitioners but heavily relied on patients' technological capabilities.[31] Another study found that 80% of patients found virtual clinic visits to be just as good as an in-person visit.[32] In sum, digital access and broadband adoption are inherently tied to usage of telehealth and present primary care providers with the impetus for having critical conversations about digital access with policymakers and patients, in addition to directly encouraging patients to seek out and use telehealth options where available.

Although the aforementioned areas—health care access and navigation, health engagement and education, and telehealth and related health behaviors—demonstrate specific ways that digital access influences patient health outcomes, it is important to note that high-quality broadband access can ultimately reduce health disparities and bridge gaps in access, information, and services for those who are underserved by systematic injustices within the health care system more broadly. Further, although digital access is important, access alone is not enough to change health outcomes for all. It is essential that health care systems, primary care providers included, understand not only their patients' digital access needs but also the larger environmental factors—digital devices and skills—that oftentimes dictate patients' digital experience and abilities.

Digital Devices and Interventions as a Social Determinant of Health

Expanding the conversation beyond digital access, patients' abilities to afford, obtain, and effectively use digital devices and digital health interventions are a key aspect of health in the digital domain. Digital devices include personal computers, smartphones, and other Internet-enabled devices (eg, smart watch, tablet), whereas digital health interventions might include watching physical therapy exercises on YouTube. Although these methods for providing health insight digitally seem accessible to many, it may not be as accessible to those who may benefit most—such as those who are low income, older adults, or those without stable housing. As with digital access, digital devices and digital health interventions can exacerbate the digital divide if not implemented with a digital equity lens. In other words, when health-related knowledge is transferred via digital health interventions and delivered via digital devices that are not fully accessible, patient health suffers as a result.[33]

Interestingly, Perakslis and Ginsburg (2020) contend that digital health technology development should be scrutinized to the same extent as other medical devices, which means that some digital health technology practices—that may lack cohesive implementation and testing for efficacy and impact—leave questions in terms of clinical validity and utility.[34] In other words, as more digital health interventions are created and put into practice, the field must continue to test both the implementation and efficacy of such practices to ensure patient use of these tools actually benefit their health. On a different note, Blease (2022) outlines the negatives that this increased, open communication via digital health technologies could have on patient perceptions of digital health interventions and their efficacy. Specifically, the phenomenon known as the "nocebo effect"—knowing too much about your care and experiencing negative outcomes based on such perceptions—could come into play as digital health interventions share increased amounts of data points and insights that patients may interpret on their own incorrectly or without support from their provider. However, when taken into consideration and intentionally addressed, providers may be able to mitigate some of these issues by helping patients to understand the role of digital health interventions as a support, not a replacement, to provider expertise and guidance.[35] These examples illustrate just some of the considerations providers must understand, as patient access to digital devices and digital health interventions increases; however, an important strategy for mitigating these challenges is described in the following section: patient digital health literacy and skills.

Digital Health Literacies and Skills as a Social Determinant of Health

Although digital access and device use are necessary precursors for patient digital health, primary care providers would be remiss to underestimate the influence of digital health literacy (eg, correcting misinformation) and digital skills (eg, digital fluency and technology navigation skills) when understanding how the digital domain influences patient health outcomes. As a reminder, digital health literacy involves the application of one's cognitive and social abilities to access, understand, and use health information within digital contexts and environments with a goal of learning about, addressing, or solving a health problem.[9] The most pressing concern for primary care providers when it comes to digital health literacy is whether their patients have the ability to understand their health records and the information about their health. Low digital health literacy not only deepens health disparities and inequalities within the landscape of an increasingly digitized health care environment but also prevents patients from engaging with the aforementioned areas of digital access (eg, EHRs, telehealth) and digital devices (eg, wearables).[36]

Correcting health misinformation

A key digital health literacy skill involves being able to distinguish credible, evidence-based health insight from misinformation shared online in formal (eg, medical websites) and informal (eg, personal blogs, chatrooms, social media) health care settings.

Further, research on health literacy rates suggests that only 12% of US adults are "proficient" or able to read and synthesize medical information and generate correct, complex insights pertinent to their health.[37] The same study found that people with disabilities make up a disproportionate number of patients with basic and below basic health literacy. In addition, the advance of social media platforms has exacerbated health misinformation online; this is especially true for information about vaccines, drugs or smoking, noncommunicable diseases, pandemics, eating disorders, and medical treatments.[38] In the end, determining the credibility of health information and finding trusted sources is crucial to health outcomes, and social media is oftentimes the culprit, not the solution. However, one study found that creating engaging and relevant patient education via YouTube videos was not only preferred by patients to traditional methods of health education but also promoted self-care practices and increased health outcomes for patients managing chronic conditions (ie, diabetes).[39] This delivery format was also viewed as being more accessible and scalable—2 important goals for providers wanting to have a greater impact when sharing evidence-based insight with patients.

At the end of the day, primary care providers plan an important role in addressing misinformation by helping patients to select digital health information that is credible and well suited for their specific needs. Doing so requires not only sharing correct health information and insight but also corrective actions, such as unpacking misinformed beliefs and teasing apart misconceptions held by patients.[40] Providers can help patients with online searches, help them to navigate online webpages, and review online sites with patients to assess for credibility, while introducing patients to practices for finding and using credible Web sites. Overall, patient-provider trust and relationship building are key for addressing misinformation over time, which presents challenges for digital health environments if patients do not communicate regularly with their providers. (Mis)information is only half the battle for digital health literacy; patients must also be fluent in using digital technology and platforms themselves.

Promoting of digital fluency

Digital fluency, or "the ability to engage with all aspects of digital technology from accessing the Internet to navigating telehealth applications, and performing basic troubleshooting," is an essential skill that in many ways drives patients' abilities to be digitally literate.[41] Key barriers to patients' digital fluency include language, age, education levels, and employment status, as well as general digital knowledge when it comes to troubleshooting issues as they arise.[41] Without being able to understand the information available on digital health platforms, patients lose interest, get frustrated, and fail to see the value that they provide. For example, a patient who has an interest in using telehealth options based on their rural location may be able to access high-quality broadband and the necessary digital devices for accessing their patient health portal. They might also be well versed in all the relevant studies about their condition and know how to ask their provider clarifying questions to avoid being misinformed. However, they might still experience digital disenfranchisement if they are not digitally fluent and have the skills to join the video telehealth conferencing platform and turn on their video to connect with and receive consultation from their doctor.

In this patient's situation, the promise of the digital equity falls short because digital skills training is oftentimes the last area of focus within the digital inclusion conversation.

In addition, many of the challenges that precede this one must be solved before the development of digital skills and fluency can even be discussed. We argue, however, that digital fluency can be the linchpin for digital health equity. Even if a patient does not yet have the necessary digital access or devices, efforts providers put forth to support patients' digital skills and fluency—which may include connecting them with a digital navigator program, digital health coach, or using a universal digital literacy screener to discern areas of growth—can further catalyze patient broadband adoption and device use by demonstrating the health value of digital health information more broadly. In other words, if patients are digitally fluent, they will feel more empowered to seek out and advocate for their rights to digital access and other health technology use.

Other Aspects of the Digital Domain

Outside of the aforementioned areas of digital equity and inclusion, primary care providers can play critical roles in 2 additional areas within the digital domain: patient health advocacy and community engagement using digital tools. Patient health advocacy focuses on addressing patient needs through frameworks that are patient-centered, coordinate care, and provide accessible services. Telemedicine and telehealth can offer ways to create those frameworks in more effective and efficient ways, although "telehealth platforms have still not been fully adapted to create a space whereby all the important advocates for a patient's health, including community health workers, behavioral health specialists, and pharmacists, interact in a way that best supports and advocates for a patient."[41(p2846)] In particular, there is a need for creating national standards for telehealth, as well as federal and state policies to support telehealth infrastructure more broadly. Primary care providers, as key drivers in the coordination of care, can provide a valuable voice in advocating for change.

Digital approaches also have the capacity to enhance community engagement within the health care system, by addressing community tech norms as well as by creating more equitable and inclusive clinical trials. Communities may have preferences for particular tools (ie, WeChat, Zoom), and understanding and supporting these community tech norms may improve adoption and engagement for specific communities.[17] Leveraging digital approaches can also strengthen community engagement with clinical trials by making it easier to recruit participants, incorporate community input, and understand the ecological contexts of participants—ultimately improving health outcomes and enhancing equity as a result.[42]

CASE STUDY

A 76-year-old woman with diabetes, heart disease, and recent stroke is wheel-chair bound. She has difficulty with transportation and mobility. She has very little family and lives in an independent living, senior high-rise. Because of her chronic illnesses, she is supposed to see you every 3 months. Her health has declined due to poor management of her diabetes and because she has missed several appointments due to lack of transportation. You note that she would benefit from telehealth visits and ask if there is anyone who can support her in connecting to the Internet and learning how to access the teleconference platform on the hospital's online portal. You make the following suggestions or referrals.

SUMMARY

Just as with more general narratives of the digital divide, digital disenfranchisement—which includes lack of digital access, devices, and skills—poses issues for health care accessibility and quality of care. Standardization of definitions of telehealth and telemedicine,[29] as well as the standardization of platforms used for digital health (including accessibility) are important for adoption and use, as well as ensuring that patients have the support they need to use new technologies fully.[41] Primary care physicians must be mindful of the ways in which digital health technologies, portals, and online communication influence the patient-provider relationship, as well as exacerbate preexisting and new health inequities as a result of digital inequities that plague society's newfound digitization of person-place-platform, as it pertains to the health care system and patient health overall.

CLINICS CARE POINTS

- Providers should keep in mind that patients may lack affordable high-quality broadband access and adoption. Providers should consider using a universal digital literacy screener to discern areas of growth for individual patients.
- When having explicit conversations with patients about new and existing technologies, providers should be aware that patients may not be comfortable or see the need for using digital health technologies and devices; others may not have access to them. This one-on-one discussion is essential, however, as discussing the ways digital access, devices, and fluency can improve patient health allows providers to build trust, encourage uptake and digital use, and discern which patients may need additional support and digital inclusion resources.
- Because digital fluency—including digital health literacy—continues to present a challenge for many patients, providers should work to connect their patients with local digital navigator programs and digital health coaches who may be able to provide more individualized assistance.
- Providers can play an important role in addressing misinformation by helping patients to select digital health information that is credible and well suited for their specific needs. Providers can also help patients with online searches, help them to navigate online webpages, and review online sites with patients to assess for credibility, while introducing patients to practices for finding and using credible Web sites.
- Systematic change—in addition to individual skills and behavior—is necessary for digital equity. As such, providers can advocate for universal digital access, support patient broadband adoption, and directly encourage the uptake and use of trusted digital health platforms that will enhance patient care.

DISCLOSURE

The authors have nothing to disclose.

REFERENCES

1. Ahern DK, Woods SS, Lightowler MC, et al. Promise of and potential for patient-facing technologies to enable meaningful use. Am J Prev Med 2011;40(5):S162–72.
2. Kickbusch I, Piselli D, Agrawal A, et al. The Lancet and Financial Times Commission on governing health futures 2030: growing up in a digital world. Lancet (British edition) 2021;398(10312):1727–76.
3. Abernethy A, Adams L, Barrett M, et al. The promise of digital health: Then, now, and the future. NAM Perspectives 2022;6(22). https://doi.org/10.31478/202206e.
4. Darkins AW, Cary MA. *Telemedicine and telehealth: Principles, policies, performance and pitfalls*. Free Association Books; 2000.

5. Ng SW, Hwong WY, Husin M, et al. Assessing the availability of teleconsultation and the extent of its use in malaysian public primary Care Clinics: Cross-sectional Study. JMIR formative research 2022;6(5):e34485.
6. Meskó B, Drobni Z, É Bényei, et al. Digital health is a cultural transformation of traditional healthcare. mHealth 2017;3:38.
7. Vogels EA, Perrin A, Raine L, Anderson M. 53% of Americans say the internet has been essential during the covid-19 Outbreak. Pew Research Center: Internet, Science & Tech. Available at: https://www.pewresearch.org/internet/2020/04/30/53-of-americans-say-the-internet-has-been-essential-during-the- covid-19-outbreak/. 2021. Accessed February 17, 2023.
8. Early J, Hernandez A. Digital disenfranchisement, and COVID-19: Broadband internet access as a social determinant of health. Health Promot Pract 2021; 22(5):605–10.
9. Yang K, Hu Y, Qi H. Digital health literacy: Bibliometric analysis. J Med Int Res 2022;24(7):e35816.
10. van Kessel R, Wong BLH, Clemens T, et al. Digital health literacy as a super determinant of health: More than simply the sum of its parts. Internet interventions: the application of information technology in mental and behavioural health 2022;27: 100500.
11. Perrin A, Atske S. 7% of Americans don't use the internet. who are they? Pew Research Center. Available at: https://www.pewresearch.org/fact-tank/2021/04/02/7-of-americans-dont-use-the-internet-who-are-they/. 2021. Accessed February 17, 2023.
12. Poon L. There are far more Americans without broadband access than previously thought. Bloomberg CityLab. Available at: https://www.bloomberg.com/news/articles/2020-02-19/where-the-u-s-underestimates-the-digital-divide. 2020. Accessed February 17, 2023.
13. Addressing social determinants of health through community research. Centers for Disease Control and Prevention. Available at: https://www.cdc.gov/prc/issue-briefs/addressing-social-determinants-of- health.html#:~:text=Social%20determinants%20of%20health%20. 2022. Accessed February 17, 2023.
14. Sieck CJ, Sheon A, Ancker JS, et al. Digital inclusion as a social determinant of health. NPJ digital medicine 2021;4(1):52.
15. Sheon A. Conference report: Digital skills: A hidden 'super' social determinant of health. IAPHS. Available at: https://iaphs.org/conference-report-digital-skills-hidden-super-social-determinant-health/. 2020. Accessed February 17, 2023.
16. Ye J, Wang Z, Hai J. Social networking service, patient-generated health data, and population health informatics: National cross-sectional study of patterns and implications of leveraging digital Technologies to support mental health and well-being. J Med Internet Res 2022;24(4):e30898.
17. Richardson S, Lawrence K, Schoenthaler AM, et al. A framework for digital health equity. NPJ digital medicine 2022;5(1):119.
18. The Words Behind Our Work: The Source for Definitions of Digital Inclusion Terms. National Digital Inclusion Alliance. Available at: https://www.digitalinclusion.org/definitions/, 2022. Accessed February 17, 2023.
19. National Broadband Map. Federal Communications Commission. Available at: https://broadbandmap.fcc.gov/home#/. Accessed February 17, 2023.
20. Bauerly BC, McCord RF, Hulkower R, et al. Broadband access as a public health issue: The role of law in expanding broadband Access and Connecting Underserved Communities for Better Health Outcomes. J Law Med Ethics 2019; 47(2_suppl):39–42.

21. Benda NC, Veinot TC, Sieck CJ, et al. Broadband internet access is a social determinant of health. Am J public health (1971) 2020;110(8):1123–5.
22. Perzynski AT, Roach MJ, Shick S, et al. Patient portals and broadband internet inequality. J Am Med Inf Assoc: JAMIA 2017;24(5):927–32.
23. Rainie L. Digital divides 2016. Pew Research Center: Internet, Science & Tech. Available at: https://www.pewresearch.org/internet/2016/07/14/digital-divides-2016/, 2020. Accessed February 17, 2023.
24. Yoose B. When libraries become medical screeners: User health data and library privacy. Choose Privacy Every Day. https://chooseprivacyeveryday.org/when-libraries-become-medical-screeners-user-health-data-and-library- privacy/. Published May 13, 2020. Accessed February 17, 2023.
25. Chan J. Exploring digital health care: eHealth, mHealth, and librarian opportunities. J Med Libr Assoc 2021;109(3):376–81.
26. Dendere R, Slade C, Burton-Jones A, et al. Patient portals facilitating engagement with inpatient electronic medical records: A systematic review. J Med Internet Res 2019;21(4):e12779.
27. Giuse NB, Koonce TY, Storrow AB, et al. Using health literacy and learning style preferences to optimize the delivery of health information. J Health Commun 2012;17(sup3):122–40.
28. Improving access to telehealth. Telehealth.HHS.gov. https://telehealth.hhs.gov/providers/health-equity-in- telehealth/improving-access-to-telehealth/. Accessed February 17, 2023.
29. Roy J, Levy DR, Senathirajah Y. Defining telehealth for research, implementation, and equity. J Med Internet Res 2022;24(4):e35037.
30. Clare CA. Telehealth and the digital divide as a social determinant of health during the COVID-19 pandemic. Network modeling and analysis in health informatics and bioinformatics (Wien) 2021;10(1). https://doi.org/10.1007/s13721-021-00300-y.
31. Burton L, Rush KL, Smith MA, et al. Empowering patients through virtual care delivery: Qualitative study with micropractice clinic patients and health care providers. JMIR formative research 2022;6(4):e32528.
32. Rose S, Hurwitz HM, Mercer MB, et al. Patient experience in virtual visits hinges on technology and the patient- clinician relationship: A large survey study with open-ended questions. J Med Internet Res 2021;23(6):e18488.
33. Jenkins CL, Imran S, Mahmood A, et al. Digital health intervention design and deployment for engaging demographic groups likely to Be affected by the digital divide: Protocol for a systematic scoping review. JMIR research protocols 2022; 11(3):e32538.
34. Perakslis E, Ginsburg GS. Digital health-the need to assess benefits, risks, and value. JAMA, J Am Med Assoc 2021;325(2):127–8.
35. Blease C. Sharing online clinical notes with patients: implications for nocebo effects and health equity. J Med Ethics 2023;49:14–21.
36. Heath S. Digital health literacy stands in the way of patient tech adoption. PatientEngagementHIT. Available at: https://patientengagementhit.com/news/digital-health-literacy-stands-in-the-way-of-patient-tech-adoption. Published April 25, 2022. Accessed February 17, 2023.
37. Newkirk C. National measures of health literacy. MSU Extension. https://www.canr.msu.edu/news/national_measures_of_health_literacy. 2018. Accessed February 17, 2023.
38. Suarez-Lledo V, Alvarez-Galvez J. Prevalence of health misinformation on social media: Systematic Review. J Med Int Res 2021;23(1):e17187.

39. Liu X, Zhang B, Susarla A, et al. Go to YouTube and see me tomorrow: Social media and self-care of chronic conditions. SSRN Electron J 2017;44(1b):257–83.
40. Schulz PJ, Nakamoto K. The perils of misinformation: when health literacy goes awry. Nat Rev Nephrol 2022;18(3):135–6.
41. Gergen Barnett K, Mishuris RG, Williams CT, et al. Telehealth's double-edged sword: Bridging or perpetuating health inequities? J Gen Intern Med: JGIM 2022;37(11):2845–8.
42. Tan RKJ, Wu D, Day S, et al. Digital approaches to enhancing community engagement in clinical trials. NPJ digital medicine 2022;5(1):37.

PART TWO: SOCIAL DETERMINANTS AND CLINICAL CARE

Social Determinants of Health, Chronic Disease Management, and the Role of the Primary Care Provider—to Include Cardiovascular Disease, Cancer, Diabetes, Major Causes of Morbidity and Mortality as Affected by Social Determinants of Health

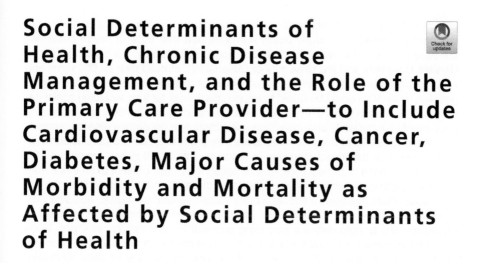

Nicholas Conley, MD

KEYWORDS

• Cortisol • Primary care provider • Diabetes • Obesity • Hypertension • Depression

KEY POINTS

- Stress can increase cortisol secretion, which can lead to and worsen diseases such as obesity, cardiovascular disease, cancer, and depression.
- Increased cortisol secretion in the morning and evening has more of an impact in a chronic disease than increased cortisol secretion during waking hours.
- Mindfulness, meditation, and exercise can reduce cortisol levels, which, if done at key intervals, may have a significant effect on health outcomes.

INTRODUCTION

Despite groundbreaking advances in medical science, pharmaceuticals, and surgical techniques, American health outcomes paradoxically continue to worsen. Primary care providers (PCPs) are on the front line of this crisis, seeing a persistent increase in number of and extent of medical comorbidities. Many physicians enter medicine with a desire to help others, but this idealism frequently gives way to frustration by lack of efficacy of their medical interventions. This frustration may not be unfounded

Cooperative Recovery, Integrated Health Cooperative at Mental Health Cooperative, 275 Cumberland Bend, Nashville TN 37228, USA
E-mail address: Nicholas.l.conley@gmail.com

Prim Care Clin Office Pract 50 (2023) 671–678
https://doi.org/10.1016/j.pop.2023.04.011
primarycare.theclinics.com

as conventional medical interventions may only be addressing a small part of health outcomes. A novel 2019 study boldly demonstrated that 60% of health outcomes are based on zip code rather than genetic code.[1,2] This study, conducted jointly by Harvard University and the University of Queensland, studied over 56,000 twins and 724,000 sibling pairs determining that only 40% of disease outcomes were linked to genetics while 60% could be linked to environmental risk factors, including social determinants of health (SDoH). In primary care, the clinician has the dual task of treating the current disease while also managing risk factors and preventing disease progression. Although some of the interventions are truly proactive, such as vaccine administration, much of traditional medicine is reactive. This tradition has grown out of a practical approach to patient care, that is, patients typically present to an office after they have a complaint and have noticed signs of disease, and not before. Over the last 2 decades, there has been a shift to a more value-centric care model, including mitigation and management of risk factors. This shift has led to a utilization of various predictive models to help define a screening protocol for disease, for example, Wells Score for predicting the likelihood of pulmonary embolus, "CHADsVASC" score for predicting the likelihood of cerebrovascular events in the face of atrial fibrillation, and so on. But, although these calculations are undeniably useful in-patient care, they are still reactive and are by definition only able to apply increased resources to those patients who are already showing signs of a disease.

The Harvard/Queensland study noted above and others[3,4] have shown that roughly half of health outcomes are dependent on factors which the US medical education has largely ignored until recently, SDoH. The first section of this article will explore the pathophysiology of how social determinants can and do create and worsen disease states. The second section will offer guidance on how the primary care provider can use this knowledge to better screen and address common diseases.

EXPLORING THE PATHOPHYSIOLOGY OF HOW SDoH CAN AFFECT DISEASE STATES

To anyone who has practiced in a resource-poor environment, the direct role of socioeconomic status on health outcomes is clear. For example, a diabetic patient whose only reliable access to nutrition is prepackaged processed food at the local gas station is clearly going to have higher blood sugar and hemoglobin A1c levels than someone who has access to affordable and fresh fruits and vegetables. Similarly, a patient who can only access salt-rich canned foods will have a higher blood pressure than the patient who has wider foods choices—an issue especially important in hypertensive patients who will see a 5- to 7-mm Hg drop in systolic blood pressure with lowered salt use.[5,6] These areas lacking fresh foods are referred to as "food deserts" and are defined by the US Department of Agriculture as areas with poverty rates greater than 20% and with greater than 33% of individuals living over a mile from a large grocery store (10 miles for rural populations).[7,8] However, there are deeper, physiologic effects that food deserts and other SDoH can have—effects due to chronically elevated stress and cortisol levels.

The English word "stress" refers to several different concepts, and the human body is often subjected to various stressors throughout the day (see the article on Vincent Morelli and Robert Joseph Heizelman article, "monitoring SDoH," in this issue for a further discussion of stress and allostatic load). In many ways, stresses are a catalyst for growth, such as carrying a heavy load causing the body to rebuild muscles and increase muscle mass or running to increase cardiac efficiency. However, stress is often accompanied by an increase in adrenal gland activity, including increase epinephrine and ultimately cortisol excretion. Practically, these processes allow for the "fight or flight" response, which can allow humans to escape dangerous environments. In these acute and brief uses, the benefits of steroid secretion far outweigh the negatives. Yet, long-term cortisol exposure is harmful and, as this article will show, forms the basis of how social determinates of health contribute to chronic disease states.

SDoH and adverse child experiences (both discussed in depth in other articles in this issue) demonstrate how stressful events such as violence, abuse, and growing up in substance use scenarios can affect health outcomes. The damages from these stressors, many of which involve the effects of cortisol, do not stop in childhood. They have cumulative effects, producing chronic cortisol-secretion states that can go on to affect health in adolescence and adulthood. Events such as violence in the community and household, working long hours, little autonomy or control of situations, poor living conditions, and exposure to the elements can all result in increased physiologic stress and cortisol secretion.[9] The hypothalamus-pituitary-adrenal axis, or HPA axis, is a well-known circular endocrine pathway which regulates many hormones secreted in the body and is particularly susceptible to cortisol response. The following sections will seek to give a brief physiologic basis for the role of stress and cortisol in forming and worsening many chronic disease states that the primary care physician will see in a typical practice.

Cortisol and Obesity

In the "fight or flight" scenario, the body needs immediate blood glucose for proper neurologic and muscle function. In chronic stress, however, elevated cortisol leads to an increase fat deposition and insulin insensitivity,[10] thus linking chronic stress exposures with obesity[11] in both animal[12] and human studies.[11] This phenomenon is seen independently of types of food consumed.[13,14] Cortisol overexpression is also tied to a decrease in expression of ghrelin and leptin, two powerful hormones in weight control and appetite suppression.[11] So, not only is someone more likely to convert blood glucose to fat in chronic stress situations, but they are also more likely, because of changes in these hormones, to eat larger portion sizes.[6] For an in-depth discussion of monitoring serum, urinary, and hair cortisol, see the article on Vincent Morelli and Robert Joseph Heizelman article, "monitoring SDoH," in this issue.

If increased cortisol caused by socioeconomic factors was only linked to obesity, then it would warrant a significant role in the discussion of health outcomes. However, the impact does not stop there. Adipose, or fat tissue itself, is considered an endocrine organ and can further increase blood sugar levels and signal insulin release, which, overtime, can lead to even greater insulin sensitivity and a higher likelihood of developing type II diabetes. Further accentuating this tendency toward diabetes is cortisol's modulation of zinc, a mineral critical in signaling insulin release[15]—again having been proven to be associated with a higher incidence of diabetes.[16]

Cortisol, Stress, Sleep, and Mental Health

In addition to cortisol's effects link to diabetes, a relationship has been identified between type 2 diabetes and circadian rhythm disruption mediated by epinephrine.[17] Increased nighttime epinephrine levels may decrease sleep quality, by way of interruption to sleep cycles and circadian rhythm. Without proper sleep, mental clarity and acuity suffers, often resulting in a decrease in mood.[18]

In this way, cortisol may also have a profound role in mental health. There has been a longstanding association between HPA axis disruption, cortisol/stress, and major depressive disorder; however, the exact role has not been well understood until recently. A 2021 meta-analysis showed an association specifically with elevated nocturnal and morning cortisol levels.[19] This showed their role as a predictive model for the onset of depression rather than a biomarker to diagnosis depression. Increased cortisol at other times of the day did not display this association. Excess cortisol will decrease other steroids, including sex hormones, also leading to a depressive effect on mood.[20] Furthermore, serotonin and dopamine levels are negatively modulated by excess cortisol secretion. This demonstrates the physiologic basis for depression in the context of stress and cortisol secretion. This physiologic basis does much to explain increased mental health disorders, including depression, in areas of health inequality and the stress induced by suboptimal SDoH. Moreover, in a 2019 cross sectional study blinded researchers were able, using physiologic data such as cortisol concentration, sleep quality, and inflammatory cytokines, to identify participants who had scored high on depression rating scales.[21] Those with the higher biomarkers also scored higher on depression rating scales.

Stress Cytokines Cortisol and the Immune Response

One such inflammatory cytokine is interleukin 1-β or IL-1β, which has been identified in antibody production; prostaglandin production; and T-cell, B-cell, and neutrophil activation (see the article on Vincent Morelli and Robert Joseph Heizelman article, "monitoring SDoH," in this issue). In addition, IL-1β has a role in signaling norepinephrine release and melatonin release.[22] IL-1β is modulated by cortisol release, and in acute stress scenarios, it produces an adaptive response promoting an immune response. However, chronic stress responses can produce a sustained and unresolved inflammatory state in which certain cell lines proliferate at the expense of others, producing an ineffective immune reponse.[23] In addition, prolonged cortisol secretion can lead to cortisol resistance, whereas cortisol will increase IL-1β rather than decrease it,[22] which will result in an imbalance between cortisol, norepinephrine, and melatonin and shift production away from TH1 (T helper cells which defend against intracellular pathogens) to TH2 (T helper cells which defend against extracellular pathogens). When cortisol is excreted for prolonged periods of time, the body's immune system slows and alters production of the beneficial immune cell lines that help to reduce tumor growth. Instead, the body increases production of selective immune cells, which may in part explain the increased rates of cancer and autoimmunity in a chronic stress state.[24]

Normally, when a cell develops uncontrolled growth, the immune system steps in and stops that growth. However, in a chronic stress state, where IL-1β increases norepinephrine and melatonin, IFNγ production is decreased, and the immune system can no longer stop that growth, and the likelihood of cancer cell proliferation is higher. In this way, sDoH not only directly increase cancer incidence through well-known environmental factors, such as cigarette smoking, but also increase the incidence of unregulated cell growth progressing to cancer by dampening the body's immune system via stress and chronic cortisol release.

Cortisol, Stress, and Cardiovascular Disease

What the primary care provider (PCP) will see in his/her practice is often the downstream effects of chronic excess cortisol, for example, the correlation between cortisol and cardiac health. As stated, cortisol influences epinephrine,[17] as well as norepinephrine modulation.[22] This can cause an increased sympathetic tone, which when combined with the chronic increase in cortisol itself that has been associated with a 2.23-times increase in prevalence of hypertension.[25] Thus, it is not in the acute stress reaction but in long-term elevated stress conditions that cardiac health is negatively affected.

A heart's efficiency, or cardiac output, is defined by heart rate multiplied by stroke volume. In times of exercise, heart rate increases but stroke volume remains constant, which increases cardiac output and allows for proper perfusion of tissues. As with any muscle, repeated use leads to changes and growth. With routine aerobic exercise, each side of the heart is subjected to increased demand: the left side from pressure to circular blood to the body, and the right side with increased pulmonary pressure from the lungs. This results in a sarcomere elongation and eccentric left ventricular hypertrophy in context of both right and left ventricular dilation.[25] Thus, the volume of the heart chamber is increased. As stroke volume is increased, the heart rate required to continue the same level of cardiac output goes down, which is why athletes develop a lower resting heart rate. In contrast, in episodes of pathologic stress, which do not involve sustained pulmonary pressures, only the left side of the heart remodels. In the context of increased vascular resistance, the heart has to pump harder to achieve the same output, and sarcomeres thicken instead of lengthening. This results in less ventricular volume, and thus, a higher heart rate is required to produce the same level of cardiac output. A feedback loop develops in which the heart continues to work harder, and more negative cardiac remodeling takes place until heart failure develops.

UTILIZING THIS KNOWLEDGE TO BETTER SCREEN AND ADDRESS COMMON DISEASES

Although extensive screening for SDoH is currently beyond the capacity of most PCPs in the US health system,[26] clinicians must still hold a high index of suspicion for these determinants. For example, the pediatric patient who presents with wheezing must be probed for SDoH as they relate to pediatric asthma—poverty,[27,28] environmental toxins,[29] and allergens such as dust mites, molds, and so on.[30–32] Other presenting complaints such as heart disease, hypertension, obesity, sleep disturbance, and mental illness should prompt similarly more extensive inquiries into SDoH and more appropriate follow-up.

The aforementioned physiologic examples demonstrate the power that cortisol, which comes from stressors, has on development of and worsening of chronic disease states. This places into context the results from the Harvard study that 60% of health outcomes are related to zip code rather than genetic code. However, all hope is not lost for those patients subjected to higher levels of stress, as these cortisol levels may be mitigated by protective factors as discussed in the article on "resilience" in this issue. PCPs can educate and recommend stress reduction techniques such as meditation, exercise, resilience training, and coping skills—all of which can help to reduce the amount of stress a body is subjected to. In addition, some PCPs may find it in their abilities to advocate for systemic changes—social programs designed to assist with income, housing, violence in the home, availability of healthy foods, education—social determinants able to ameliorate the deleterious effects of stress.

As stated, although it is beyond the practical scope of most physician practices to incorporate many such larger scale changes, as stated above, there is a distinct role for primary care physicians to screen for stress patterns (SDoH) and intervene to improve health outcomes. Mindfulness and meditation can be introduced by PCPs and have been shown to reduce cortisol levels.[33,34] (Social media and video platforms, such as YouTube, can help as most patients have easy and free access to high-quality mindfulness and meditation courses via these tools.) PCPs may also recommend and discuss ways to best incorporate low-impact aerobic exercise—also linked to cortisol reduction—into patient lifestyles. As with mindfulness, there is a plethora of free and easy-to-use instructional videos for yoga on YouTube and other social media sites. Yoga does not involve costly equipment and can be practiced in small spaces, making it ideal for patients who do not have access to safe areas to walk or run. The low-impact nature of yoga also allows patients with joint disease, obesity, or the elderly to engage in this form of exercise. Indeed, incorporating opportunities for mindfulness, low-impact aerobic exercise, and sleep hygiene are just a few simple ways that PCPs can help reduce stress levels, cortisol levels, and play a significant role in mitigating many of the disease states discussed in this article.

If 60% of health outcomes are indeed linked to SDoH, then that would suggest that 60% of current health disparities could be mitigated by changing social determinants. Thus, an effective way of treating an overburdened and struggling health care system in this country would be to decrease the number of chronic diseases by improving environmental factors such as SDoH. Although many of these changes are outside of the scope of the PCP, needing to come from policy changes at the local, state, and national levels, the PCP can engage with patients to identify and reduce stress levels. Using education, therapeutic resources, appropriate referrals, and opportunities provided through technology, providers can effect positive health outcomes to a far greater degree than current best practices can alone.

CLINICS CARE POINTS

- Comprehensive social history should be performed on each patient as social determinants of health effect primary care outcomes.
- When treating diabetes, heart disease, and obesity, consider reviewing social stressors with your patient.
- Consider low-cost, widely available interventions such as mindfulness and meditation as ways to reduce stress in patients.

DISCLOSURES

The author has nothing to disclose.

REFERENCES

1. Lakhani CM, Tierney BT, Manrai AK, et al. Repurposing large health insurance claims data to estimate genetic and environmental contributions in 560 phenotypes. Nat Genet 2019;51:327–34.
2. Tomiyama AJ. Stress and Obesity. Annu Rev Psychol 2019;70:703–18.
3. Hood CM, Gennuso KP, Swain GR, et al. County health rankings: relationships between determinant factors and health outcomes. Am J Prev Med 2016;50: 129–35.
4. Mackenbach JP. The contribution of medical care to mortality decline: McKeown revisited. J Clin Epidemiol 1996;49:1207–13.
5. He FJ, MacGregor GA. Effect of longer-term modest salt reduction on blood pressure. Cochrane Database Syst Rev 2004;3:CD004937.
6. He FJ, Li J, Macgregor GA. Effect of longer term modest salt reduction on blood pressure: Cochrane systematic review and meta-analysis of randomised trials. BMJ 2013;346:f1325.
7. Available at: https://www.ers.usda.gov/amber-waves/2011/december/data-feature-mapping-food-deserts-in-the-us/.

8. Available at: https://www.cdc.gov/pcd/issues/2014/14_0086.htm.
9. Bremner JD. Traumatic stress: effects on the brain. Dialogues Clin Neurosci 2006; 8(4):445–61.
10. Geiker NRW, Astrup A, Hjorth MF, et al. Does stress influence sleep patterns, food intake, weight gain, abdominal obesity and weight loss interventions and vice versa? Obes Rev 2018;19(1):81–97.
11. Van der Valk ES, Savas M, van Rossum EFC. Stress and Obesity: Are There More Susceptible Individuals? Curr Obes Rep 2018;7(2):193–203.
12. Morais JBS, Severo JS, Beserra JB, et al. Association Between Cortisol, Insulin Resistance and Zinc in Obesity: a Mini-Review. Biol Trace Elem Res 2019; 191(2):323–30.
13. Hewagalamulage SD, Lee TK, Clarke IJ, et al. Stress, cortisol, and obesity: a role for cortisol responsiveness in identifying individuals prone to obesity. Domest Anim Endocrinol 2016;56(Suppl):S112–20.
14. Salehi M, Ferenczi A, Zumoff B. Obesity and cortisol status. Horm Metab Res 2005;37(4):193–7.
15. Gumus Balikcioglu P, Balikcioglu M, Soros A, et al. The 24-hour average concentration of cortisol is elevated in obese African-American youth with type 2 diabetes. J Diabetes Complications 2021;35(7):107933.
16. Giessner S, Ramaker ME, Blew K, et al. Disrupted Circadian Rhythm of Epinephrine in Males With Youth-Onset Type 2 Diabetes. J Endocr Soc 2022;7(2): bvac190.
17. Zajkowska Z, Gullett N, Walsh A, et al. Cortisol and development of depression in adolescence and young adulthood - a systematic review and meta-analysis. Psychoneuroendocrinology 2022;136:105625.
18. Walker MP. The role of sleep in cognition and emotion. Ann N Y Acad Sci 2009; 1156:168–97.
19. Chronister BN, Gonzalez E, Lopez-Paredes D, et al. Testosterone, estradiol, DHEA and cortisol in relation to anxiety and depression scores in adolescents. J Affect Disord 2021;294:838–46.
20. Jia Y, Liu L, Sheng C, et al. Increased Serum Levels of Cortisol and Inflammatory Cytokines in People With Depression. J Nerv Ment Dis 2019;207(4):271–6 [Erratum in: J Nerv Ment Dis. 2019;207(7):610].
21. Zefferino R, Di Gioia S, Conese M. Molecular links between endocrine, nervous and immune system during chronic stress. Brain Behav 2021;11(2):e01960.
22. Maes M, Van der Planken M, Stevens WJ, et al. Leukocytosis, monocytosis and neutrophilia: hallmarks of severe depression. J Psychiatr Res 1992;26(2):125–34.
23. Bautista LE, Bajwa PK, Shafer MM, et al. The relationship between chronic stress, hair cortisol and hypertension. Int J Cardiol Hypertens 2019;2:100012.
24. Dai S, Mo Y, Wang Y, et al. Chronic Stress Promotes Cancer Development. Frontiers in oncology 2020;10:1492.
25. Fulghum K, Hill BG. Metabolic Mechanisms of Exercise-Induced Cardiac Remodeling. Front Cardiovasc Med 2018;5:127.
26. Friedman S, Caddle S, Motelow JE, et al. Improving Screening for Social Determinants of Health in a Pediatric Resident Clinic: A Quality Improvement Initiative. Pediatr Qual Saf 2021;6(4):e419.
27. Harris KM. Mapping inequality: Childhood asthma and environmental injustice, a case study of St. Louis, Missouri. Soc Sci Med 2019;230:91–110.
28. Osman M, Tagiyeva N, Wassall HJ, et al. Changing trends in sex specific prevalence rates for childhood asthma, eczema, and hay fever. Pediatr Pulmonol 2007; 42:60.

29. Influence of Rural Environmental Factors in Asthma - Jennilee Luedders 1, Jill A Poole. Immunol Allergy Clin North Am 2022;42(4):817–30. https://doi.org/10.1016/j.iac.2022.05.008.
30. Matsui EC, Abramson SL, Sandel MT, et al. Indoor Environmental Control Practices and Asthma Management. Pediatrics 2016;138.
31. De Vera MJ, Drapkin S, Moy JN. Association of recurrent wheezing with sensitivity to cockroach allergen in inner-city children. Ann Allergy Asthma Immunol 2003; 91:55.
32. Perry T, Matsui E, Merriman B, et al. The prevalence of rat allergen in inner-city homes and its relationship to sensitization and asthma morbidity. J Allergy Clin Immunol 2003;112:346.
33. Pascoe MC, Thompson DR, Ski CF. Yoga, mindfulness-based stress reduction and stress-related physiological measures: A meta-analysis. Psychoneuroendocrinology 2017;86:152–68.
34. Pascoe MC, Thompson DR, Jenkins ZM, et al. Mindfulness mediates the physiological markers of stress: Systematic review and meta-analysis. J Psychiatr Res 2017;95:156–78.

Social Determinants of Mental and Behavioral Health

Leigh Morrison, MD*, Christopher J. Frank, MD, PhD

KEYWORDS

- Social determinants • Mental health • Mental illness

KEY POINTS

- Both mental health and mental illness are impacted by social determinants.
- The absence of serious mental illness does not guarantee optimal mental health.
- Social prescribing is a tool available to primary care clinicians to link patients with appropriate social and community services to address sub-optimal social determinants of mental health.
- Caring for children's mental and behavioral health includes screening and treating mental and behavioral health issues in parents/caretakers.
- Randomized controlled trials are needed to test scalable interventions designed to improve mental health and minimize the impact of mental illness.

HISTORY AND BACKGROUND

The underlying causes and mechanisms of poor mental health and serious mental illness are an unsolved mystery. From divine punishment or invasion by evil spirits, to disruptions in bodily fluids, imbalances of yin and yang, the Biblical consequence of drinking undiluted wine, the impact of excessive masturbation, and myths about the impact of a "wandering" womb, the one great constant of mental illness is the search for an explanation.[1]

The discovery in the early twentieth century that infection by *Treponema pallidum* was the cause of neurosyphilis (general paresis of the insane), raised hopes that mental illnesses could be explained by single causes.[2] But simple causes and clear treatments for other mental illnesses remained elusive.

In 1909, the mental hygiene movement began in the United States with a goal of preventing mental illness. This movement believed that the root causes of many mental illnesses were environmental – being raised in a dangerous neighborhood or by bad

Department of Family Medicine, University of Michigan
* Corresponding author. 300 North Ingalls Street, NI4C06, Ann Arbor, MI 48109-5435.
E-mail address: morrisol@med.umich.edu

Prim Care Clin Office Pract 50 (2023) 679–688
https://doi.org/10.1016/j.pop.2023.04.003
primarycare.theclinics.com
0095-4543/23/

parents. Soldiers returning from both World Wars with *shell shock* or *war neurosis* demonstrated that exposure to trauma could lead to profoundly impaired mental health.[2]

In the mid-20th century, the social psychiatry movement drew on ecological studies in Chicago and New Haven showing that individuals with serious mental illnesses were disproportionately concentrated in poor neighborhoods and that mental illness was not evenly distributed across social classes.[3]

In 1963, President Kennedy spoke of the need to "seek out the causes of mental illness and of mental retardation and eradicate them." Of those causes, he drew the most attention to "harsh environmental conditions."[3] While twin studies, genetic linkages and medication treatments have solidified our understanding of the role that genetics play in mental illness, it is clear that our environment and life experiences, or "social determinants," contribute to both serious mental illness (SMI) and mental health in general.

SMI and mental health are often lumped together when talking about the social determinants of mental health (SDOMH). The World Health Organization defines mental health as "a state of mental well-being that enables people to cope with the stresses of life, realize their abilities, learn well and work well, and contribute to their community."[4] SMI usually refers to disorders such as schizophrenia, bipolar disorder, and major depression, that can have profound impacts on function. But even in the absence of an SMI, mental health is not a guarantee.

The SDOMH are qualitatively similar to the social determinants of physical health.[5] Fundamentally, these determinants are due to the unequal distribution of opportunity as influenced by public policies and social norms leading to stress, restricted choices, high-risk behaviors, and the associated physical and mental health fallout.[6,7]

PREVALENCE AND INCIDENCE

SDOMH can be divided into discreet categories, although for individuals and communities they are often intertwined.[6] Most people affected by suboptimal social determinants of health are affected by many determinants at once. For organizational ease, we will describe the association of *individual* social determinants of health with mental health and mental illness.

Racial Discrimination and Social Exclusion

Discrimination and social exclusion are associated with negative mental health outcomes. Experiencing racism in infancy and early childhood adversely impacts socioemotional and behavioral development.[8] The vast majority of African American (90%) and Afro-Caribbean (87%) teenagers have experienced discrimination, and discrimination in these groups was associated with increased lifetime rates of anxiety and depression.[9] In adolescents and adults, racial discrimination has been associated with psychosis, mood disorders, and anxiety disorders.[10] Discrimination toward multiracial people appears to be on a continuum, with those receiving the highest level of discrimination reporting the worst mental health outcomes, including anxiety and depression.[11] Minority status plays a significant role when considering the intersectionality between race and sexual orientation. Specifically, minority youth who have been marginalized due to sexual orientation and gender identity have higher rates of suicide.[12] And among people identifying as a sexual minority, those exposed to discrimination based on sexual identity are more likely to have psychiatric disorders and substance use disorders.[13] The prevalence of substance use is 2.5 to 4 times higher for transgender youth compared to their non-transgender peers.[14] Like other excluded groups with suboptimal social determinants of health, immigrants often integrate lower on the social gradient in their new country of residence and have worse mental health outcomes.[15]

Adverse Early Life Experiences

Adverse early life experiences including family violence, neglect, or abuse are associated with a range of psychiatric symptoms[16] including post-traumatic stress disorder,[17] and the development of substance use disorders in adulthood.[18] Emotional abuse as a child is an important predictor of future psychiatric symptoms.[19]

Poor Education and Neighbor Deprivation

Poor educational environments at home and school can impact long-term mental health outcomes. The home literacy environment is positively impacted by higher parental socioeconomic status and maternal education and is negatively impacted by maternal depression.[20] In the school system, children learn important psychological and social skills, and children who struggle to develop these skills are more prone to depression, anxiety, and feelings of hopelessness, helplessness, and worthlessness.[6] School is also a resource for screening and early intervention for common learning and mood disorders. Schools in poorer communities often have lower quality instruction, higher student-to-teacher ratios, and fewer academic resources, which can negatively impact cognitive, social, and language development.[20] Language impairment is associated with increased risk of attention deficit hyperactivity disorder, affective disorders, and anxiety disorders.[20]

Poverty, Unemployment, Job Insecurity, and Income Inequality

Poverty, debt, and income inequality are associated with mental illness and poor mental health.[21,22] Among youth ages 10 to 15, the prevalence of depressed mood or anxiety was reported to be 2.5x higher in youth with low socioeconomic status compared to age-matched peers with higher socioeconomic status.[23] Among working age adults, involuntary job loss is associated with increased risk and severity of depression and anxiety, and unemployed people report high levels of uncertainty about the future, anger, shame, and loss of self-esteem after job loss.[24,25] The duration of unemployment appears to have a cumulative effect on psychological distress, with those unemployed longer having higher relative risk of suicide.[26] Conversely, job security and a sense of control at work are protective factors for mood disorders.[27,28]

Poor Housing Quality, Housing Instability, and the Built Environment

The quality and stability of housing plays an important role in mental health. The structural features of the home (eg, multi-unit dwelling, higher floor level, high-risk apartment building) are associated with depression among women.[29] Overcrowding can lead to increased stress at home and family violence.[30] Conversely, individuals who rate their housing environments more favorably report less psychiatric distress and better residential satisfaction and adaptive functioning.[31]

Poor Access to Sufficient Healthy Food

Food insecurity is associated with depression and anxiety, with a dose-response relationship between the severity of food insecurity and the prevalence of depressive symptoms.[32] Mechanistically, food insecurity seems to lead to a psychological stress response which is associated with poor social development in children,[6] lower student grade point average and poorer mental health in college students,[33] and higher levels of anxiety, frustration, and a sense of powerlessness in adults.[6] Individuals with food insecurity tend to buy lower-cost, energy-dense, processed foods, which can have negative impacts on development in infants and school-aged children and long term impacts on both physical and mental health.[6]

THERAPEUTIC OPTIONS

There is limited evidence to guide how best to identify and address the SDOMH, but they are so intertwined with poor mental health and mental illness that mental health concerns should trigger an exploration of the life experiences and environment of the patient. For primary care physicians, using a short, pragmatic, and validated screening tool to identify SDOMH is one option.[34] The American Academy of Family Physicians provides both short- and long-form screening tools, as well as a Social Determinants of Health (SDOH) Patient Action Plan.[35] To promote honest disclosure, self-administered tests are favored over in-person interviews, particularly for sensitive information such as interpersonal violence.[36] Supplemental mood and substance use questionnaires (eg, Patient Health Questionnaire-9, Generalized Anxiety Disorder-7, National Institute on Drug Abuse Quick Screen) can be used in conjunction with SDOH screening tools to assess mental health.

Social prescribing is one technique for addressing SDOMH identified by screening.[6,7,25,34,37] Social prescribing is a network function in which patients are linked to appropriate social and community services, or more intensive health care services.[25] The approach should be collaborative, sharing tasks between specialists, generalists, and community members, including social service organizations.[25] Case management is central to this approach, and improves both mental and physical health outcomes in people with comorbid mental and physical conditions, as well as improving satisfaction with care and promoting better quality of life.[25] Given the shortage of mental health care resources in the United States, many primary care physicians may be forced to rely on models that intensify services based on disease severity and trajectory. In resources-scarce settings, a step model can be used where low-cost, low-intensity interventions are used for patients with mild symptoms, and care is intensified if symptoms plateau or worsen.[25] Studies have shown that this approach improves mental health outcomes in the primary care setting.[38,39] An example is a collaborative care model with a community mental health center where supportive housing may only be available when patients have a qualifying SMI and severe disability.

To better understand disparities in mental health, it is important to understand how these disparities are generated both transgenerationally and over an individual lifespan.[40] This life course model posits that current health "is shaped by earlier exposures (even decades before) to physical, environmental, and psychosocial factors."[40] **Fig. 1** provides a schematic look at the life course model as developed by the World Health Organization.

Linking the social determinants of mental health with the life course model can help prioritize interventions on programs that impact multiple parts of the life course. For example, the prenatal and early years periods are heavily influenced by adverse early life experiences and poor education. One adverse early life experience is having a caregiver with prenatal, perinatal, or maternal depression, which not only impacts parents but also impacts cohabitating children. Screening for and treating maternal depression can improve mental health outcomes for both parents and children.[41,42] Extensive evidence supports multiple *home visiting programs* that focus on families with infants and demonstrate improved outcomes in a range of SDOMH including reductions in abuse and neglect,[43] maternal depression,[41] and improvements in short-term developmental outcomes and long-term social and behavioral outcomes in enrolled children.[44,45]

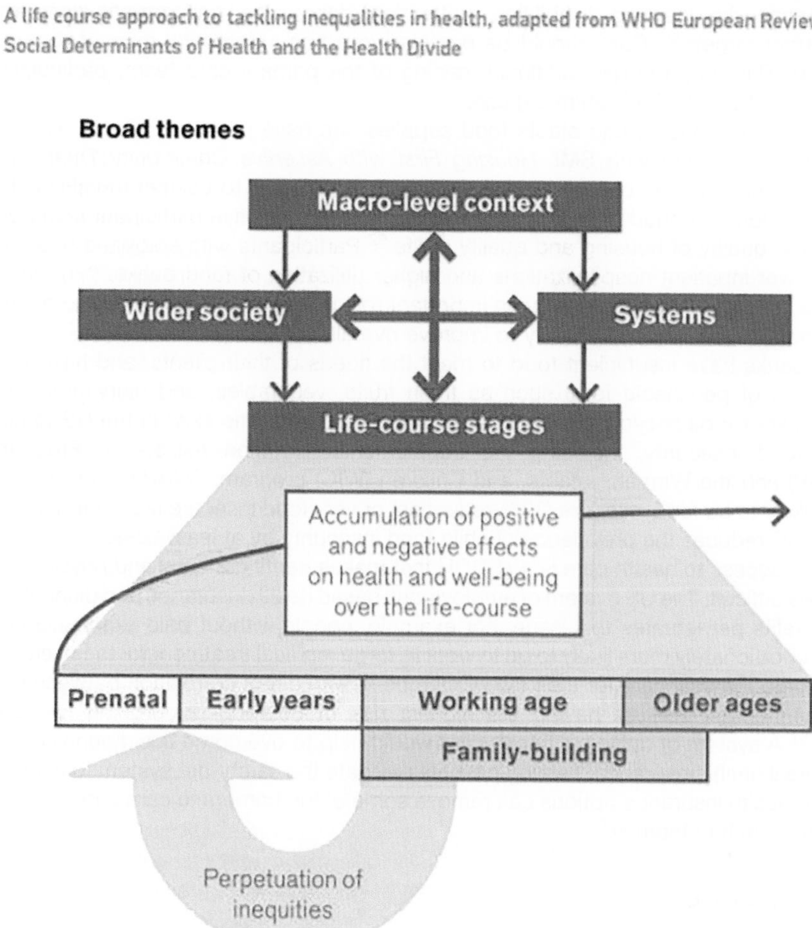

Fig. 1. The life course model. (*From* World Health Organization and Calouste Gulbenkian Foundation. Social determinants of mental health. Geneva, World Health Organization, 2014.)

During childhood, *early education programs* can improve the social determinants of mental health and high-quality preschools improve educational attainment at older ages.[46] The High/Scope Perry Preschool Program increased intelligent quotients (IQ $\geq$ 90) at age five, graduation rates from high school, income at age 40, and also decreased criminal justice involvement.[47,48] In the US, clinicians can refer children and low-income parents to the Head Start and Early Head Start programs for both educational services and social and nutritional services for the family. Parental engagement in reading improves outcomes and early literacy programs that focus on parental involvement such as Reach Out and Read, or book gifting programs (eg, Dolly Parton's Imagination Library) can improve outcomes.[49]

For *parents with substance use disorders*, case management and appropriate referral to a higher level of care increases recovery rates and helps prevent child abuse and neglect.[50] Globally, mental and substance use disorders account for one-quarter of years lived with disability in children and youth, making early identification of substance use, learning disabilities, inattention, depression, and anxiety disorders important targets.[51] Care should be provided in a non-judgmental manner, free of stigma. This may require additional training of the primary care team, particularly when practicing LGBTQ-affirming care.

Permanent housing and stable food supplies can have profound effects on outcomes for patients with SMI. *Housing First with Assertive Community Treatment (ACT) programs* have been extremely successful in leading to quicker transitions to housing, longer periods spent in stable housing, and a positive participant rating on both the quality of housing and quality of life.[52] Participants with stabilized housing had fewer inpatient hospitalizations and higher utilization of food banks.[53] In terms of food stability, food banks play an important role in relieving immediate food deprivation, but have limited capacity to improve overall food security outcomes.[54] Most food banks have insufficient food to meet the needs of their clients, and have low amounts of perishable food such as fresh fruits, vegetables, and dairy products necessary for balanced nutritional needs.[54] Several programs exist in the US to aid with food insecurity, including the Supplemental Nutrition Assistance Program (SNAP) and the Women, Infants, and Children (WIC) program. SNAP recipients are less likely to be food insecure (30% reduction) or very food insecure (20% reduction), and WIC reduces the prevalence of child food insecurity by at least 20%.[55,56]

Poor access to health care is an SDOH that makes treating mental and physical illnesses difficult. The US system of employment-based health insurance and disparities in benefits perpetuates this issue. For example, people without paid sick leave are disproportionately more likely to go to work ill, forgo medical treatment for themselves, and forgo medical care for their family members, with direct correlation between the lowest-income workers having the highest risk of delaying or forgoing medical care.[57] A system of universal health care would help to overcome this. Even without universal health insurance, helping patients navigate the safety-net system to access public health insurance options can remove some of the barriers to care and improve mental health outcomes.[58]

CONTROVERSIES

The general principle that mental health and mental illness are impacted by our environment and experience seems so basic as to be boring. What we know about the social determinants of both physical and mental health are mostly from association studies. This presents a challenge for designing interventions because targeting root causes often depends on understanding causal relationships, something that association studies often cannot answer.

Screening for SDOMH may be a useful approach to guide social prescribing, but like other screening tests that depend on access to an effective treatment, in most communities we do not know if screening improves outcomes. And even when interventions are successful in small studies and controlled environments (eg, Perry Preschool Study), it can be a challenge to scale these interventions.

The US health care system currently lacks a broad social safety net to address the wide range of social determinants of mental and physical health. Until a widespread cultural change that prioritizes equity and inclusivity takes hold, we will need to selectively evaluate interventions to identify the most impactful programs. The SDOMH are complicated and intertwined, and the reality that some interventions will not work or are not scalable, is not a reason to stop building future programs that might prove beneficial. Modern medicine is peppered with examples of programs that make intuitive sense but do not hold up in rigorous studies. Because the SDOMH touch all parts of the social fabric, there are almost unlimited options for designing programs that might work. Randomized trials and sophisticated observational studies will need to help identify the best new interventions, but scaling up interventions that already work (like home visiting programs) are an opportunity to start shifting public resources toward prevention.

SUMMARY AND FUTURE DIRECTIONS

Finally, as primary care clinicians, we must acknowledge the reciprocal impact of poor mental health and mental illness on the social determinants of mental health. Poor mental health and mental illness are associated with homelessness, school dropout, marital instability, and economic insecurity.[59] Mental illness affects living and employment conditions, which limit opportunities for upward mobility on the social gradient.[59] However, the slope of the social gradient is not fixed, and addressing social stratification and inequitable access to opportunities, especially in early life, may allow for improvement in the social determinants of health and ultimately lessen mental illness and improve mental health.[5,60]

CLINICS CARE POINTS

- There is a wide variety of evidence-based programs that improve mental health outcomes.
- Social prescribing is a tool available to primary care clinicians to link patients with appropriate social and community services to aid in addressing sub-optimal social determinants of mental health.
- Caring for children's mental and behavioral health includes screening and treating mental and behavioral health issues in parents/caretakers.
- Screening for social determinants of mental health only works when effective interventions are available.
- One approach to promote equity is to focus resources and interventions on the most severely disadvantaged individuals, and communities and families with children.

DISCLOSURE

The authors have nothing to disclose.

REFERENCES

1. Scull A. Madness in civilization: a cultural history of insanity, from the bible to Freud, from the madhouse to modern medicine. Princeton, NJ: Princeton University Press; 2015.
2. Harrington A. Mind fixers: psychiatry's troubled search for the biology of mental illness. 1st edition. New York, NY: W.W. Norton & Company; 2019.
3. Smith M. An ounce of prevention. Lancet 2015;386(9992):424–5.
4. Mental health: strengthening our response Available at: https://www.who.int/news-room/fact-sheets/detail/mental-health-strengthening-our-response. Accessed December 19, 2022.
5. Marmot M, Friel S, Bell R, et al. Closing the gap in a generation: health equity through action on the social determinants of health. Lancet 2008;372(9650):1661–9.

6. Compton MT, Shim RS. The Social Determinants of Mental Health. American Psychiatric Publishing; 2014. Available at: http://ebookcentral.proquest.com/lib/umichigan/detail.action?docID=5515112. Accessed September 5, 2022.
7. Compton MT, Shim RS. The Social Determinants of Mental Health. FOCUS 2015;13(4):419–25.
8. Berry OO, Londoño Tobón A, Njoroge WFM. Social Determinants of Health: the Impact of Racism on Early Childhood Mental Health. Curr Psychiatry Rep 2021;23(5):23.
9. Pachter LM, Caldwell CH, Jackson JS, et al. Discrimination and Mental Health in a Representative Sample of African-American and Afro-Caribbean Youth. J Racial Ethn Health Disparities 2018;5(4):831–7.
10. Berger M, Sarnyai Z. More than skin deep": stress neurobiology and mental health consequences of racial discrimination. Stress 2015;18(1):1–10.
11. Franco M, Durkee M, McElroy-Heltzel S. Discrimination comes in layers: Dimensions of discrimination and mental health for multiracial people. Cultur Divers Ethnic Minor Psychol 2021;27(3):343–53.
12. Estimating the Risk of Attempted Suicide Among Sexual Minority Youths: A Systematic Review and Meta-analysis | Adolescent Medicine | JAMA Pediatrics | JAMA Network. Available at: https://jamanetwork-com.proxy.lib.umich.edu/journals/jamapediatrics/fullarticle/2704490. Accessed September 17, 2022.
13. Lee JH, Gamarel KE, Bryant KJ, et al. Discrimination, Mental Health, and Substance Use Disorders Among Sexual Minority Populations. LGBT Health 2016;3(4):258–65.
14. Day JK, Fish JN, Perez-Brumer A, et al. Transgender Youth Substance Use Disparities: Results From a Population-Based Sample. J Adolesc Health Off Publ Soc Adolesc Med 2017;61(6):729–35.
15. Hynie M. The Social Determinants of Refugee Mental Health in the Post-Migration Context: A Critical Review. Can J Psychiatry Rev Can Psychiatr 2018;63(5):297–303.
16. Kessler RC, McLaughlin KA, Green JG, et al. Childhood adversities and adult psychopathology in the WHO World Mental Health Surveys. Br J Psychiatry 2010;197(5):378–85.
17. Mohammad ET, Shapiro ER, Wainwright LD, et al. Impacts of Family and Community Violence Exposure on Child Coping and Mental Health. J Abnorm Child Psychol 2015;43(2):203–15.
18. Oladeji BD, Makanjuola VA, Gureje O. Family-related adverse childhood experiences as risk factors for psychiatric disorders in Nigeria. Br J Psychiatry 2010;196(3):186–91.
19. Cecil CAM, Viding E, Fearon P, et al. Disentangling the mental health impact of childhood abuse and neglect. Child Abuse Negl 2017;63:106–19.
20. Perkins SC, Finegood ED, Swain JE. Poverty and Language Development: Roles of Parenting and Stress. Innov Clin Neurosci 2013;10(4):10–9.
21. Jenkins R, Bhugra D, Bebbington P, et al. Debt, income and mental disorder in the general population. Psychol Med 2008;38(10):1485–93.
22. Lund C, Breen A, Flisher AJ, et al. Poverty and common mental disorders in low and middle income countries: A systematic review. Soc Sci Med 2010;71(3):517–28.
23. Lemstra M, Neudorf C, D'Arcy C, et al. A Systematic Review of Depressed Mood and Anxiety by SES in Youth Aged 10–15 Years. Can J Public Health 2008;99(2):125–9.

24. Catalano R, Goldman-Mellor S, Saxton K, et al. The health effects of economic decline. Annu Rev Public Health 2011;32:431–50.
25. Barry MM, Clarke AM, Petersen I, et al, editors. Implementing mental health promotion. Switzerland AG: Springer Nature; 2019. https://doi.org/10.1007/978-3-030-23455-3.
26. Milner A, Page A, LaMontagne AD. Cause and effect in studies on unemployment, mental health and suicide: a meta-analytic and conceptual review. Psychol Med 2014;44(5):909–17.
27. Esser I, Olsen KM. Perceived Job Quality: Autonomy and Job Security within a Multi-Level Framework. Eur Sociol Rev 2012;28(4):443–54.
28. Bambra C, Egan M, Thomas S, et al. The psychosocial and health effects of workplace reorganisation. 2. A systematic review of task restructuring interventions. J Epidemiol Community Health 2007;61(12):1028–37.
29. Evans GW, Wells NM, Moch A. Housing and Mental Health: A Review of the Evidence and a Methodological and Conceptual Critique. J Soc Issues 2003;59(3): 475–500.
30. The Impact of Overcrowding on Health and Education: A Review of the Evidence and Literature. Office of the Deputy Prime Minister; 2004.
31. Wright PA, Kloos B. Housing environment and mental health outcomes: A levels of analysis perspective. J Environ Psychol 2007;27(1):79–89.
32. Leung CW, Epel ES, Willett WC, et al. Household Food Insecurity Is Positively Associated with Depression among Low-Income Supplemental Nutrition Assistance Program Participants and Income-Eligible Nonparticipants. J Nutr 2015; 145(3):622–7.
33. Martinez SM, Frongillo EA, Leung C, et al. No food for thought: Food insecurity is related to poor mental health and lower academic performance among students in California's public university system. J Health Psychol 2020;25(12):1930–9.
34. Jeste DV, Pender VB. Social Determinants of Mental Health: Recommendations for Research, Training, Practice, and Policy. JAMA Psychiatr 2022;79(4):283–4.
35. 2019 - Guide to social needs screening.pdf. Available at: https://www.aafp.org/dam/AAFP/documents/patient_care/everyone_project/hops19-physician-guide-sdoh.pdf. Accessed November 29, 2022.
36. Gottlieb L, Hessler D, Long D, et al. A Randomized Trial on Screening for Social Determinants of Health: the iScreen Study. Pediatrics 2014;134(6):e1611–8.
37. Bickerdike L, Booth A, Wilson PM, et al. Social prescribing: less rhetoric and more reality. A systematic review of the evidence. BMJ Open 2017;7(4):e013384.
38. Araya R, Rojas G, Fritsch R, et al. Treating depression in primary care in low-income women in Santiago, Chile: a randomised controlled trial. Lancet 2003; 361(9362):995–1000.
39. Patel V, Weiss HA, Chowdhary N, et al. Effectiveness of an intervention led by lay health counsellors for depressive and anxiety disorders in primary care in Goa, India (MANAS): a cluster randomised controlled trial. Lancet 2010;376(9758): 2086–95.
40. Jones NL, Gilman SE, Cheng TL, et al. Life Course Approaches to the Causes of Health Disparities. Am J Public Health 2019;109(Suppl 1):S48.
41. Rahman A, Malik A, Sikander S, et al. Cognitive behaviour therapy-based intervention by community health workers for mothers with depression and their infants in rural Pakistan: a cluster-randomised controlled trial. Lancet 2008; 372(9642):902–9.

42. Patel V, Chisholm D, Parikh R, et al. Addressing the burden of mental, neurological, and substance use disorders: key messages from Disease Control Priorities, 3rd edition. Lancet. 2016;387(10028):1672-1685.
43. Olds DL. Long-term effects of home visitation on maternal life course and child abuse and neglect. Fifteen-year follow-up of a randomized trial. JAMA 1997; 278(8):637–43.
44. Barnes J, MacPherson K, Senior R. The impact on parenting and the home environment of early support to mothers with new babies. J Child Serv 2006; 1(4):4–20.
45. Sowden AJ, Tilford S, Delaney F, et al. Mental health promotion in high risk groups. Qual Health Care 1997;6(4):219–25.
46. Melhuish EC, Sylva K, Sammons P, et al. Preschool Influences on Mathematics Achievement. Science 2008;321(5893):1161–2.
47. Schweinhart LJ, Montie J, Xiang Z, et al. The High/Scope Perry Preschool Study Through Age 40. Ypsilanti, MI: High/Scope Press; 2005. p. 194–215.
48. Belfield CR, Nores M, Barnett S, et al. The High/Scope Perry Preschool Program: Cost-Benefit Analysis Using Data from the Age-40 Followup. J Hum Resour 2006; 41(1):162–90.
49. Full Text. Available at: https://journals.sagepub.com/doi/pdf/10.3102/0034654320922140. Accessed January 9, 2023.
50. Grant TM, Ernst CC, Streissguth A, et al. Preventing Alcohol and Drug Exposed Births in Washington State: Intervention Findings From Three Parent-Child Assistance Program Sites. Am J Drug Alcohol Abuse 2005;31(3):471–90.
51. Erskine HE, Moffitt TE, Copeland WE, et al. A heavy burden on young minds: the global burden of mental and substance use disorders in children and youth. Psychol Med 2015;45(7):1551–63.
52. Aubry T, Goering P, Veldhuizen S, et al. A Multiple-City RCT of Housing First With Assertive Community Treatment for Homeless Canadians With Serious Mental Illness. Psychiatr Serv Wash DC 2016;67(3):275–81.
53. Kerman N, Sylvestre J, Aubry T, et al. The effects of housing stability on service use among homeless adults with mental illness in a randomized controlled trial of housing first. BMC Health Serv Res 2018;18(1):190.
54. Bazerghi C, Mckay FH, Dunn M. The Role of Food Banks in Addressing Food Insecurity: A Systematic Review. J Community Health 2016;41(4):732–40.
55. Ratcliffe C, McKernan SM. How Much Does Snap Reduce Food Insecurity? :32.
56. Kreider B, Pepper JV, Roy M. Identifying the Effects of WIC on Food Insecurity Among Infants and Children. South Econ J 2016;82(4):1106–22.
57. Workers Without Paid Sick Leave Less Likely To Take Time Off For Illness Or Injury Compared To Those With Paid Sick Leave | Health Affairs. Available at: https://www.healthaffairs.org/doi/10.1377/hlthaff.2015.0965. Accessed September 29, 2022.
58. McMorrow S, Gates JA, Long SK, et al. Medicaid Expansion Increased Coverage, Improved Affordability, And Reduced Psychological Distress For Low-Income Parents. Health Aff 2017;36(5):808–18.
59. Alegría M, NeMoyer A, Falgàs Bagué I, et al. Social Determinants of Mental Health: Where We Are and Where We Need to Go. Curr Psychiatry Rep 2018; 20(11):95.
60. Marmot M, Bell R. Social inequalities in health: a proper concern of epidemiology. Ann Epidemiol 2016;26(4):238–40.

PART THREE: RESILIENCE

Resilience and Sub-optimal Social Determinants of Health

Fostering Organizational Resilience in the Medical Profession

Mekeila C. Cook, MS, PhD[a,*], Ruth Stewart, MD[b,c]

KEYWORDS

• Resilience • Social determinants of health • Medical school • Residency training
• Organizational resilience

KEY POINTS

- The aftermath of the COVID-19 pandemic highlighted the necessity for organizational resilience in health care.
- Distinguishing resilience from well-being and self-care can elevate individual and community resiliency building as an essential tool for improving the outcomes of the healthcare workforce.
- We suggest building resilience through medical training and reviewing current curriculum and clinical practice.

DEFINING RESILIENCY

Resilience, described as a process than a personal characteristic or trait, is the ability to adapt and thrive despite adversity.[1] Scholars explain that resilience is "the negotiation, management and adaptation to significant stress and/or trauma".[2,3] Research on resilience typically focuses on the environment or the individual and originates in the fields of ecology and psychology. In ecology, resilience is defined as "a measure of how much disturbance an ecosystem can endure without shifting to a different state".[4] In the early years of psychology, resilience was observed via longitudinal

[a] Division of Public Health Practice, School of Graduate Studies and Research, Meharry Medical College, 1005 Dr. DB Todd Jr. Boulevard, Clay Simpson, Suite 213, Nashville, TN 37208, USA; [b] Department of Family and Community Medicine, Meharry Medical School, 1005 Dr. DB Todd Jr. Boulevard, Nashville, TN 37208, USA; [c] Department of Professional and Medical Education, Meharry Medical School, 1005 Dr. DB Todd Jr. Boulevard, Nashville, TN 37208, USA
* Corresponding author.
E-mail address: mcook@mmc.edu

Prim Care Clin Office Pract 50 (2023) 689–698
https://doi.org/10.1016/j.pop.2023.04.013

studies and focused on identifying protective and at-risk factors that either benefited or hindered individual growth.[4] In this article, we describe the relationship between resilience and social determinants of health (SDOH) and how medical training can infuse resiliency within the curriculum and clinical practice. We will use the case study of Jessica[1] to illustrate the ways in which resilience can manifest at the individual level as well as community and organizational opportunities to foster resilience.

The Case of Jessica

Jessica was 9 when she was diagnosed with acute lymphoblastic leukemia. She lived in a rural area without access to a hospital, so she traveled 90 minutes away from her family home for treatment. Jessica experienced many of the complications that can arise from chemotherapy, and she spent many weeks in the hospital while receiving chemotherapy and being treated for complications from the chemotherapy. Jessica's parents worked to afford health insurance, so she spent many hours alone or with her grandmother while receiving treatment. Jessica's community rallied around her parents during treatment and provided funds for travel and time off of work. In addition, several people from the community volunteered to care for the family home, doing yard work and caring for the pets, so Jessica's parents could be with her during treatment as much as possible when they were off of work.

Jessica enjoyed being in the hospital when she thought well enough to play and interact with the staff, nurses, and doctors. She asked a lot of questions, proved to be a quick learner, and was encouraged to think about a career in medicine when she grew older. After 2 years of arduous treatment, Jessica was in remission, and started routine posttreatment care. As a middle schooler, Jessica excelled in school, told everyone she was going to be a doctor, and joined 4-H to improve her communication and skill set to help her get ready for college. No one in her family had ever been to college, and she only knew that colleges liked to see community involvement and extracurricular activities on applications.

Jessica graduated at the top of her class in high school, attended state college on loans and scholarships, and worked hard to get into medical school. Her MCAT scores were lower than hoped for, and she was denied admission the first time she applied. After college graduation, she returned to her hometown, took a job in a local pharmacy as a pharmacy technician, and resumed studying for the MCAT. Her second application cycle was successful, and she was admitted to the state medical school several hours away from her family.

Jessica performed well in medical school and matched into her top choice family medicine program in another state. While in residency, her father died after a short illness with brain cancer. Her residency program did not reach out or help her during her father's illness or death. In addition, she missed too much time away from the program while caring for her father at the end of his life to finish on cycle. Jessica became depressed, disillusioned with medical training and angry at herself that she had traveled so far from her hometown to train, thus leaving her mother to cope with her father's death alone. During her grief and disappointment, her romantic partner of several years ended their engagement. Because of her difficulties with worsening sleep, mood, and functioning, Jessica fell behind in documenting her medical records, was late to rounds and clinic several times, and was judged to have demonstrated "insubordination" to her program director. She was placed on probational status and advised to enter therapy, which she did, but found it minimally beneficial.

Despite these setbacks, Jessica successfully finished her training program and entered practice in community health back in her home state. She established new colleagues and friends, found a romantic partner, married, and had 2 children. Jessica worked hard to establish a wide net of support so she would not think the isolation and loss of hope she had thought during her medical training. She worked hard to establish good practice habits to ensure she kept in control of her medical records and established a good record of professional and cordial conduct.

Jessica, seeing her own journey through many difficulties, thought empowered to do what she had always longed to do, open her own medical practice. She found the right space, rehabilitated the space to create a warm and welcoming environment, hired an exceptional business manager, and opened her own practice with a clearly defined goal of caring for her community while making a living to help support her family. She used creative marketing and good business practices to grow her practice, hired additional support staff and an additional physician. A medical student who spent their family medicine clerkship with Jessica recently wrote her a thank you note expressing their admiration for "how easy you make it all look." Jessica had to chuckle. None of it had been easy, most of it had been difficult, but she recognized she had stuck with it, set realistic goals, and learned to thrive.

Leveraging the Community to Foster Resilience

Research on SDOH posits that the community people live in affects their overall health and well-being. The World Health Organization defines SDOH as "the nonmedical factors that influence health outcomes. They are the conditions in which people are born, grow, work, live, and age, and the wider set of forces and systems shaping the conditions of daily life".[5] Relatedly, community resilience is defined as the ability of a collective group of people to work together to overcome common adversity that affects people who live and work together. A related concept, collective efficacy, is defined as the mutual trust and willingness to intervene for the common good of the greater community.[6] Sampson postulated that when communities have trust with their neighbors, they are able to leverage support and resources that act as a protective factor for the community during times of adversity. In Jessica's case, when she was battling cancer, her family garnered support from their community. Neighbors offered to help care for their home and pets in their absence. They also provided financial assistance for the needs of the family. Collective efficacy is evident in the community assistance Jessica's family received during her years of treatment. The community's willingness, ability, and responsiveness to Jessica and her family contributed to Jessica's individual level of resilience as well as the community's resilience.

Similarly, research investigating the environmental factors associated with SDOH that either reinforce or diminish resilience focuses on 4 key attributes: (1) inclusion, (2) social conditions, (3) access, and (4) involvement.[7] Inclusion embraces, accepts, and makes room for all genders, races, ethnicities, ages, cultures, and identities. Creating inclusive environments promotes a sense of belonging, equity, and fairness, and removes social barriers.[7] Inclusion as an environmental factor bolsters resilience. Inclusion is exemplified in Jessica's case by how she was treated by the clinical staff when she was receiving chemotherapy. The staff, nurses, and doctors entertained her inquisitiveness, answered her questions, and encouraged her to pursue a career in medicine, thus making her think a part of the team. Jessica carried these experiences with her throughout primary and secondary school.

The second factor, social conditions, relates to socioeconomic factors that directly contribute to SDOH.[5] Social conditions include having adequate and safe housing, equitable education, and appropriate medical coverage.[7] Both of Jessica's parents worked full-time jobs to ensure she had the medical coverage needed to pay for her chemotherapy. Having to work long hours resulted in Jessica being alone often or in the care of her grandmother while in the hospital. Social factors such as having appropriate medical coverage play a significant role in resilience and directly affect mental health, which is a key resource in developing resiliency.

Access is the third environmental factor attributed to resilience. Access includes the ability and resources to draw upon the health, education, and civic systems in ways that are beneficial to the individual and community. For Jessica's family, the nearest hospital that offered the treatment she required was 90 miles away from her home. The distance created significant hardship for her family to ensure she received proper care. The closure of several hospitals in rural communities in recent years has contributed to reduced access to care and health equity.[8] Health care facilities that are strategically placed for accessibility, and responsive civic systems that work together to provide residents with quality care enhance community resilience.

The final environmental factor affecting resilience is involvement. Involvement differs from inclusion in that involvement requires action on the part of the individual, whereas inclusion creates social space for all people. Active involvement not only builds self-confidence, but it also helps to expand one's community and social connections and contributes to collective efficacy. In Jessica's adult years, she sought to build her social network in a way that provided the necessary support to her during difficult times. Her proactive approach to involvement mediated the poor mental health and isolation she thought during her residency and reinforced a sense of belonging, all of which support resiliency. Jessica fostered community and through her social network, contributed to community resilience. The case study illustrates how each of the environmental factors is interconnected and follows a social gradient fashioned along socioeconomic inequity.

COVID-19 Unearths Lack of Organizational Resilience

Much of the literature on resilience focuses on the individual's ability to activate resilience, which has been touted as an answer to many social ills. Although this is an important approach, individual-level efforts should not be the primary focus for developing resilience. The concepts of community resilience can be scaled up and applied to organizations, particularly in the health care system.

Following the COVID-19 pandemic, the US public health system began the lengthy process of identifying the resiliency needs of its workforce that expand beyond disaster preparedness to consider ways to bolster workforce resilience. What is evident from the strain placed on the health care system and the clinical staff during the pandemic is the woeful conditions in which hospitals and health care facilities offered mental health care and support to their clinicians and staff.[9] The medical profession has important decisions to make to not only stay current with contemporary workforce support observed in peer countries but to also provide the necessary support for an industry facing serious and possibly catastrophic staffing shortages.[10,11] Medical schools have a duty to prepare their students with the clinical tools to offer optimal care. Where training wanes is in assisting trainees to develop the resilience skills needed to provide proper care to their patients while simultaneously caring for their own well-being.[12]

Medical Student and Resident Physician Wellness and Resiliency

Over the last several decades, the need to improve the well-being of medical students, residents, and practicing physicians has been recognized. The recent emphasis on student and resident trainee wellness in curriculum and training is due to several decades of surveys of medical students and residents demonstrating that trainees often experience a decline in their mental health throughout training, including higher incidents of anxiety, depression, burnout, self-harm, and suicidality than their same-aged peers.[13,14]

Both credentialing bodies that set the curriculum content standards, the Liaison Committee on Medical Education (LCME) for medical school and the Accreditation Council for Graduate Medical Education (ACGME) for residency, require a curriculum on wellness and mental health to address these concerns. In addition, the LCME and ACGME have standards on workload and fairness of evaluations and feedback to ensure trainees have access to clear practices and processes and leave time for personal wellness (LCME standard 8.8 and ACGME Common Program Requirements VI.C). Although it is still being determined if workload limits and required education on wellness and mental health improve student and resident outcomes, the benefits of meeting the accreditation standards may be washed out by many other factors. Other factors include the lack of workplace autonomy, financial strain due to poor compensation, student loan burden, and experiencing what some refer to as the "moral injury" of caring for patients in a health care system poorly equipped to support health care workers and their care for patients.

One common theme of well-being is having (being given or making) time for self-care. Resilience is mentioned as naturally flowing from self-care, as if there is a bank of resiliency, and the way to fill it is with self-care. In many trainings for students, residents, and practicing physicians, there is little recognition of resilience as the potential everyone brings from their lived experience is specific to an individual's life and circumstances and is built upon intentional practice rather than self-care. Emphasizing resilience is not to devalue self-care, which can be used to improve a sense of well-being. Self-care can include time away from work, pursuing outside interests and hobbies, sleep, rest, and rejuvenation through recreation. However, a distinction should be made between self-care and resilience. Self-care and well-being are not always assessable due to difficult circumstances beyond our control (eg, a health crisis, natural disasters, pandemics, and the loss of loved ones). In addition, self-care usually requires resources that include time, money, energy, and agency.

In contrast, resilience can be fostered and built with readily available resources. For example, in the above case study, Jessica was expected to return to a demanding residency program after her father's death, and there was no time for "self-care." However, what could have changed Jessica's residency outcome, and avoided the disciplinary action that placed Jessica and her career in medicine in a precarious position, was support from her program and colleagues, thus potentially bolstering Jessica's resilience and helping her overcome her professional and personal setbacks. One brief meeting with the program director after Jessica returned from her bereavement could have identified what support Jessica needed to return to her program successfully. Jessica describes this residency experience as "ostracizing and highly traumatic." Moreover, although she wishes she had never experienced the setback, she recognizes it as giving her extraordinary empathy for patients who struggle to perform (work, school, and family life) in adverse environments because of not having the community and family support that would make the difference between setbacks and successful navigation of difficulties.

In addition, distinguishing resilience from well-being and self-care can elevate individual and community resilience building as an essential tool for improving the outcomes of the health care workforce and the patients they care for. Teaching health care workers to recognize their resilience and the resilience of their patients and communities emphasizes existing and potentially emerging strengths. These strengths are the foundation for growth than depending on individual self-care banks that are filled and quickly depleted.

System Change and Improving Workplace Culture to Address Wellness and Resiliency

Mental health and wellness curricula differ across training programs, but in general, they center around reminding trainees about good habits to stay mentally healthy with self-care and how to seek help if mental health or problem behaviors become a barrier to success for the trainee, especially as it relates to their functioning in school or residency. Well-being is a complex phenomenon, and there is yet to be strong evidence that the current curricula improve student and resident well-being. Currently, the studies exploring curricula effectiveness often look at short-term measures, have fewer participants, and have limited follow-up. In addition, the curricular interventions vary widely between schools and programs, making comparisons and conclusions elusive.[15] The ACGME wellness program brings workplace culture and systemic changes to training to the forefront as potentially meaningful ways to improve wellness in trainees. Similarly, the LCME emphasizes stringent attention to clear and enforced policies, such as duty hours policies and policies guiding adequate independent study time, to promote improved medical education environments with sufficient time for study and engagement in self-care. This emphasis on systemic changes as important foundational aspects of individual and workforce wellness is an encouraging sign that the superficial emphasis on an individual's path to wellness (often with "token" offers such as chair massages, meditation sessions, lunch break yoga, and "surprise" gifts of desserts) will diminish because calls for systemic changes become more unified.

Despite the efforts of the LCME and individual medical school wellness programs, some survey data suggest that student wellness, defined as "having eight dimensions: intellectual, emotional, physical, social, occupational, financial, environmental, and spiritual"[16] has declined recently. The COVID-19 pandemic and the social isolation this might have caused, more significant societal upheaval, friend and family poor health and death, increased patient needs and demands, and even poor enforcement of work hour limits are potential contributors to this decline. Meanwhile, schools and training programs are revisiting their wellness curricula to combat the rising numbers of trainees with depression, anxiety, and other mental health concerns. Addressing resiliency awareness and training is an emerging theme to reinvigorate wellness programs, including the AAMC (Association of American Medical Colleges) program.

Adding resilience awareness and training among medical trainees is a solid step that will allow individuals to build their skills and understanding, improve their outcomes, and share and promote these skills with their patients. However, again, the caution is to ensure this training is coupled with empowering trainees to advocate for changes that further increase individual and institutional resiliency. Returning to Jessica and her difficulty in residency, it is important to revisit that it would be minimally helpful to encourage Jessica to be resilient in the face of her father's death as the residency program was unwilling to think carefully about supporting their resident and colleague through a challenging time in her life. Resiliency curricula could be offensive to students and trainees if they do not include how these individuals will be supported by resilient communities and institutions. Just as teaching patients how to recognize and use their resilience is not to replace advocating and replacing systems of oppression and dehumanizing policies and cultural practices, teaching medical trainees the same skills is not a substitute for pressing for policies that result in improving the environment and culture of medical education and residency training.

Impacting Patient Outcomes by Screening for Resiliency in Patients with Less-Than-Optimal Social Determinants of Health

As students, residents, physicians, and others on the health care team learn and intentionally enhance their individual, community, and organizational resiliency, a natural extension is to ensure patient care is placed in the context of understanding the patient in terms of individual and community resiliency. In the past, primary care physicians were trained to focus on the medical problem lists and note SDOH as contributors to poor health outcomes and part of the social history. Primary care evidence-based preventive health screenings improve patient outcomes.[17] However, SDOH often becomes the most significant predictor of overall patient quality of life and longevity.[18] Health care workers are usually only in the position of mitigating SDOH by treating the results of chronic diseases and managing these diseases' ravages on well-being, function, and longevity. In communities with less than optimal SDOH, community and societal change would have a much more significant impact on overall health and longevity than the individual treatment choices a provider makes about an individual patient's resulting chronic health problems. However, positive social and community changes are usually incremental at best. Advocating for change and effective policy for a broader impact is separate from most primary care physicians' training.

Primary care physicians have the opportunity to deliver additional impact by helping their patients identify personal characteristics and lived histories that can contribute to resiliency. Brief assessments and interventions can help the physician and the patient better understand the facilitators of resiliency and identify community measures that can contribute to resilience. For example, Jessica, given her family's history of needing help during her illness and recovery, recognizes how important extended family, community, and local resources are to her patient and the patient's family when she diagnoses her new patient with multiple myeloma. The integration of primary care and behavioral health care in clinical settings is one example of the medical field's role in bolstering patient resiliency. Medical social workers providing support beyond medical needs in pediatric units, maternal care wards, and family medicine play an essential role in delivering comprehensive patient-centered care.

Most of the recommendations for screening and patient education in primary care revolve around the search for previously undiagnosed disease states (eg, screening tools for major depressive disorder, type 2 diabetes, and hyperlipidemia), with the hope that diagnosing these conditions early will mitigate the impact of these conditions. As many providers who work in communities with less than optimal SDOH can attest, the screening and diagnosis of diseases made more frequent and deadlier by high levels of poverty and other societal ills can be akin to putting out a raging fire by ladling small spoons of water on the flames. The bigger problem is the societal, political, and cultural harms that light the match and add the accelerator to the causative factors of these chronic disease states.[19] Screening for SDOH that can improve the quality of life and longevity could be a step toward more rational screening for communities with less than optimal SDOH. Screening and offering interventions for building resilience can improve patient health and well-being, which can reduce the disease burden of communities with less than optimal SDOH. Despite being weary of the demands of mandated screenings and incremental chronic disease management, primary care physicians who embrace a tool meant to "flip the script" to screening for prior adaptations made by the patient during times of adversity can be built upon to mitigate disease progression and poor outcomes.

Providers who follow screening guidelines often use screening tools embedded in the electronic health record, and completing the screening is then used to assess the quality of care patients receive. When available in resource-strained systems, medical teams, including para-nursing staff (medical assistants and noncertified or licensed health care staff), nurses, social workers, and others, ensure the recommended screening is performed. Given the evidence for the positive impact building resiliency can have on mitigating, avoiding, and getting through future adversity, adding a validated resiliency screening tool to patient populations with less-than-optimal SDOH will help identify patients who need further assessment and referral to resiliency-building training and interventions. As with other screening tools, this could be performed by the members of the nonphysician medical team, thereby not adding undue burden to the overall cost or time of the medical encounter.

Screening patients for their ability to adapt to adversity will also place this factor in its proper place as a significant contributor to well-being and longevity. Funding, developing, and supporting resiliency-building interventions for patients and communities who need them the most is essential work, providing the framework for the necessary step beyond screening. The health coaching model already uses patient empowerment and recognition of strengths to build a patient-centered and patient-derived plan for improving outcomes. Health coaching skills, including resiliency screening and building, ideally taught early in the medical career, can be reinforced throughout training in simulated patient experiences, case-based learning, and clerkship experiences so that the recognition and building of a patient's resiliency become an assessed portion of the patient interaction while in training. Many practicing physicians already offer brief interventions based on the health coaching model (eg, tobacco cessation). These interventions can be billed for and reimbursed, especially in models that pay for high-value care.

SUMMARY

The development of resilience skills is necessary not only for the benefit of medical students and residents but also for the benefit of their patients. The organizational position on resilience has a profound impact on standard operating procedures in the practices of its clinical staff as well as in the way it provides care to its patients.

Given the aftermath of the COVID pandemic and the impact it had on clinical personnel and patients seeking care, the medical profession can seize the moment and bolster the overall wellbeing of its workforce. The World Health Organization issued several organizational recommendations to better support health care workers. Some recommendations include ensuring staffing levels that are appropriate for the flow of patients, allocating equitable workloads, providing breaks and time off between shifts, supportive supervision, and paid leave off.[12]

In addition to organizational support, there is a need for a systematic shift that prioritizes the health and well-being of health professionals. International health organizations posit that "it is the mandated obligation to protect workers through the prevention of harmful physical or mental stress due to conditions of work and to recognize the right of everyone to a world of work free from violence and harassment, including gender-based violence and harassment."[12] The WHO further suggests that it is the duty of the overall health care system to prevent harm from the dangers and hazards of its workforce by providing mental health support and protection from violence, including workplace bullying. The health care system needs to provide support with fair and equitable compensation and social protection, promote inclusivity and belonging in a safe work environment free from discriminatory practices, and finally safeguard workers' rights to collective bargaining and ensure an environment free from retaliation.

CLINICS CARE POINTS

- Addressing resiliency awareness and training is an emerging theme to reinvigorate wellness programs, including the AAMC program.
- When adding resilience awareness to medical training, ensure this training is coupled with empowering trainees to advocate for changes that further increase individual and institutional resiliency.
- When working with patients, trainees should screen for SDOH that can improve quality of life and longevity.
- Screening and offering interventions for building resilience can improve patient health and well-being, which can reduce the disease burden of communities with less than optimal SDOH.

DISCLOSURE

The authors have nothing to disclose.

REFERENCES

1. Morelli V. Adolescent health screening: an update in the age of big data. In: Morelli V, editor. *Screening for resilience in adolescents*. Elsevier; 2019. p. 191–206. https://doi.org/10.1016/C2018-0-00181-4.
2. Windle G. What is resilience? A review and concept analysis. Rev Clin Gerontol 2011;21(2):152–69.
3. Langeland Krista S, Manheim David, McLeod Gary, et al. How civil institutions build resilience: organizational practices derived from academic literature and case studies. RAND Corporation; 2016. Available at: http://www.jstor.org/stable/10.7249/j.ctt1btc0m7.
4. Kulig JC, Edge DS, Townshend I, et al. Community resiliency: Emerging theoretical insights. J Community Psychol 2013;41:6.
5. World Health Organization. Social determinants of health. Updated 2023. Available at: https://www.who.int/health-topics/social-determinants-of-health#tab=tab_1. Accessed January 5, 2023.
6. Sampson RJ, Raudenbush SW, Earls F. Neighborhoods and violent crime: a multilevel study of collective efficacy. Science 1997;277(5328):918–24.
7. Barankin T. and Khanlou N., *Growing up Resilient: ways to build resilience in children and youth*, Centre for Addiction and Mental Health, 2007. Available at: https://camh.ca/-/media/files/guides-and-publications/2887-growupresil_ins-pdf.pdf. Accessed March 1, 2023
8. American Hospital Association. Rural hospital closures threaten access: Solutions to preserve care in local communities. Updated September 30, 2022. Available at: https://www.aha.org/system/files/media/file/2022/09/rural-hospital-closures-threaten-access-report.pdf. Accessed January 30, 2023.

9. Søvold LE, Naslund JA, Kousoulis AA, et al. Prioritizing the Mental Health and Well-Being of Healthcare Workers: An Urgent Global Public Health Priority. Front Public Health 2021;9:679397.
10. American Hospital Association. Data brief: Health care workforce challenges threaten hospitals' ability to care for patients. Updated October, 2021 https://www.aha.org/system/files/media/file/2021/11/data-brief-health-care-workforce-challenges-threaten-hospitals-ability-to-care-for-patients.pdf. Accessed January 30, 2023.
11. Strategies to mitigate healthcare personnel staffing shortages. Centers for Disease Control and Prevention; 2020. Available at: https://www.cdc.gov/coronavirus/2019-ncov/hcp/mitigating-staff-shortages.html. Accessed March 25, 2023.
12. Hill MR, Goicochea S, Merlo LJ. In their own words: stressors facing medical students in the millennial generation. Med Educ Online 2018;23(1):1530558.
13. Mata DA, Ramos MA, Bansal N, et al. Prevalence of Depression and Depressive Symptoms Among Resident Physicians: A Systematic Review and Meta-analysis. JAMA 2015;314(22):2373–83.
14. Klein HJ, McCarthy SM. Student wellness trends and interventions in medical education: a narrative review. Humanit Soc Sci Commun 2022;9:92.
15. Nikolis L, Wakim A, Adams W, et al. Medical student wellness in the United States during the COVID-19 pandemic: a nationwide survey. BMC Med Educ 2021; 21(1):401.
16. Hostetter J, Schwarz N, Klug M, et al. Primary care visits increase utilization of evidence-based preventative health measures. BMC Fam Pract 2020;21(1):151.
17. Whitman A., De Lew N., Chappel A., et al., Addressing social determinants of health: examples of successful evidence-based strategies and current federal efforts, 2022, Office of Health Policy. Available at: https://aspe.hhs.gov/sites/default/files/documents/e2b650cd64cf84aae8ff0fae7474af82/SDOH-Evidence-Review.pdf. Accessed March 3, 2023.
18. Cockerham WC, Hamby BW, Oates GR. The Social Determinants of Chronic Disease. Am J Prev Med 2017;52(1S1):S5–12.
19. Abdul Rahim HF, Fendt-Newlin M, Al-Harahsheh ST, et al. Our duty of care: a global call to action to protect the mental health of health and care workers. Doha, Qatar: World Innovation Summit for Health; 2022.

UNITED STATES POSTAL SERVICE®

Statement of Ownership, Management, and Circulation (All Periodicals Publications Except Requester Publications)

1. Publication Title	2. Publication Number	3. Filing Date
PRIMARY CARE: CLINICS IN OFFICE PRACTICE	044 – 690	9/18/2023
4. Issue Frequency	5. Number of Issues Published Annually	6. Annual Subscription Price
MAR, JUN, SEP, DEC	4	$277.00

7. Complete Mailing Address of Known Office of Publication *(Not printer) (Street, city, county, state, and ZIP+4®)*
ELSEVIER INC.
230 Park Avenue, Suite 800
New York, NY 10169

Contact Person
Malathi Samayan
Telephone *(Include area code)*
91-44-4299-4507

8. Complete Mailing Address of Headquarters or General Business Office of Publisher *(Not printer)*
ELSEVIER INC.
230 Park Avenue, Suite 800
New York, NY 10169

9. Full Names and Complete Mailing Addresses of Publisher, Editor, and Managing Editor *(Do not leave blank)*

Publisher *(Name and complete mailing address)*
DOLORES MELONI ELSEVIER INC.
1600 JOHN F KENNEDY BLVD. SUITE 1600
PHILADELPHIA, PA 19103-2899

Editor *(Name and complete mailing address)*
TAYLOR HAYES, ELSEVIER INC.
1600 JOHN F KENNEDY BLVD. SUITE 1600
PHILADELPHIA, PA 19103-2899

Managing Editor *(Name and complete mailing address)*
PATRICK MANLEY, ELSEVIER INC.
1600 JOHN F KENNEDY BLVD. SUITE 1600
PHILADELPHIA, PA 19103-2899

10. Owner *(Do not leave blank. If the publication is owned by a corporation, give the name and address of the corporation immediately followed by the names and addresses of all stockholders owning or holding 1 percent or more of the total amount of stock. If not owned by a corporation, give the names and addresses of the individual owners. If owned by a partnership or other unincorporated firm, give its name and address as well as those of each individual owner. If the publication is published by a nonprofit organization, give its name and address.)*

Full Name	Complete Mailing Address
WHOLLY OWNED SUBSIDIARY OF REED/ELSEVIER, US HOLDINGS	1600 JOHN F KENNEDY BLVD. SUITE 1600 PHILADELPHIA, PA 19103-2899

11. Known Bondholders, Mortgagees, and Other Security Holders Owning or Holding 1 Percent or More of Total Amount of Bonds, Mortgages, or Other Securities. If none, check box → ☐ None

Full Name	Complete Mailing Address
N/A	

12. Tax Status *(For completion by nonprofit organizations authorized to mail at nonprofit rates) (Check one)*
The purpose, function, and nonprofit status of this organization and the exempt status for federal income tax purposes:
☒ Has Not Changed During Preceding 12 Months
☐ Has Changed During Preceding 12 Months *(Publisher must submit explanation of change with this statement)*

13. Publication Title		14. Issue Date for Circulation Data Below	
PRIMARY CARE: CLINICS IN OFFICE PRACTICE		JUNE 2023	
15. Extent and Nature of Circulation		Average No. Copies Each Issue During Preceding 12 Months	No. Copies of Single Issue Published Nearest to Filing Date
a. Total Number of Copies *(Net press run)*		70	72
b. Paid Circulation *(By Mail and Outside the Mail)*	(1) Mailed Outside-County Paid Subscriptions Stated on PS Form 3541 (Include paid distribution above nominal rate, advertiser's proof copies, and exchange copies)	51	51
	(2) Mailed In-County Paid Subscriptions Stated on PS Form 3541 *(Include paid distribution above nominal rate, advertiser's proof copies, and exchange copies)*	0	0
	(3) Paid Distribution Outside the Mails Including Sales Through Dealers and Carriers, Street Vendors, Counter Sales, and Other Paid Distribution Outside USPS®	8	10
	(4) Paid Distribution by Other Classes of Mail Through the USPS (e.g., First-Class Mail®)	10	10
c. Total Paid Distribution *[Sum of 15b (1), (2), (3), and (4)]* ▶		69	71
d. Free or Nominal Rate Distribution *(By Mail and Outside the Mail)*	(1) Free or Nominal Rate Outside-County Copies included on PS Form 3541	2	1
	(2) Free or Nominal Rate In-County Copies Included on PS Form 3541	0	0
	(3) Free or Nominal Rate Copies Mailed at Other Classes Through the USPS (e.g., First-Class Mail)	0	0
	(4) Free or Nominal Rate Distribution Outside the Mail *(Carriers or other means)*	0	0
e. Total Free or Nominal Rate Distribution *(Sum of 15d (1), (2), (3) and (4))*		2	1
f. Total Distribution *(Sum of 15c and 15e)* ▶		70	72
g. Copies not Distributed *(See Instructions to Publishers #4 (page #3))* ▶		0	0
h. Total *(Sum of 15f and g)*		70	72
i. Percent Paid *(15c divided by 15f times 100)* ▶		97.86%	98.61%

* If you are claiming electronic copies, go to line 16 on page 3. If you are not claiming electronic copies, skip to line 17 on page 3.

16. Electronic Copy Circulation	Average No. Copies Each Issue During Preceding 12 Months	No. Copies of Single Issue Published Nearest to Filing Date
a. Paid Electronic Copies ▶		
b. Total Paid Print Copies (Line 15c) + Paid Electronic Copies (Line 16a) ▶		
c. Total Print Distribution (Line 15f) + Paid Electronic Copies (Line 16a) ▶		
d. Percent Paid (Both Print & Electronic Copies) (16b divided by 16c × 100) ▶		

☒ **I certify that 50% of all my distributed copies (electronic and print) are paid above a nominal price.**

17. Publication of Statement of Ownership
☒ If the publication is a general publication, publication of this statement is required. Will be printed in the DECEMBER 2023 issue of this publication. ☐ Publication not required.

18. Signature and Title of Editor, Publisher, Business Manager, or Owner
Malathi Samayan - Distribution Controller *Malathi Samayan* Date 9/18/2023

I certify that all information furnished on this form is true and complete. I understand that anyone who furnishes false or misleading information on this form or who omits material or information requested on the form may be subject to criminal sanctions (including fines and imprisonment) and/or civil sanctions (including civil penalties).

Printed and bound by CPI Group (UK) Ltd, Croydon, CR0 4YY
03/10/2024
01040474-0003